Home
Health
Care

GERIATRIC CASE PRACTICE TRAINING SERIES

Series Editor
Joel Leon, *George Washington University*

The **Geriatric Case Practice Training Series** is designed to help students and professionals who work directly with the elderly and their families develop necessary skills and knowledge across a wide range of service settings included in the continuum of care. Each volume will examine a particular practice setting and focus on the nature of the typical client populations, problems, and service needs.

In this series...

GERIATRIC CASE PRACTICE IN NURSING HOMES
Susan O. Mercer, J. Dianne Garner, and Joel Leon

HOSPICE CARE
Bert Hayslip, Jr. and Joel Leon

HOME HEALTH CARE
Lenard W. Kaye

Forthcoming...

COMMUNITY-BASED PRACTICE
Joel Leon, Monika White, and Lynn Goldus

ACUTE-MEDICAL CARE AND ASSESSMENT
Nancy Morrow-Howell, Enola Proctor, and Joel Leon

Home Health Care

Lenard W. Kaye

Geriatric Case Practice Training Series 2
Series Editor, JOEL LEON

SAGE Publications
International Educational and Professional Publisher
Newbury Park   London   New Delhi

For information address:

SAGE Publications, Inc.
2455 Teller Road
Newbury Park, California 91320

SAGE Publications Ltd.
6 Bonhill Street
London EC2A 4PU
United Kingdom

SAGE Publications India Pvt. Ltd.
M-32 Market
Greater Kailash I
New Delhi 110 048 India

Printed in the United States of America

Library of Congress Cataloging-in-Publication Data

Kaye, Lenard W.
Home health care / Lenard W. Kaye.
        p.   cm.   —(Geriatric case practice training series; v. 2)
    Includes bibliographical references and index.
    ISBN 0-8039-2903-X (cl).   — ISBN 0-8039-2904-8 (pb)
    1. Home care services.   2. Aged—Home care.   I. Title.
II. Series.
    [DNLM: 1. Home Care Services.   W1 GE456G v. 2]
RA645.3.K39   1992
362.1'4—dc20   92-19444

92 93 94 95   10 9 8 7 6 5 4 3 2 1

Sage Production Editor: Diane S. Foster

To my wife, Susan
and my best friends, Fletcher, Tessa, and "the boys"
My sources of inspiration, support,
and uncompromising love

Contents

Preface

Home health care is one of the fastest-growing aspects of the health care industry. There is a continual demand for appropriately trained personnel. This volume serves as an introduction to the psychosocial skills and knowledge practitioners need to have to work effectively with the elderly in the home health care setting. The skills include such activities as the assessment of needs and the development of treatment plans. The knowledge base includes an understanding of the organizational nature of home health agencies and the recognition of the importance policy plays in their operation and how policies affect the delivery of care. The volume also contains model fieldwork assignments in the appendix. These model learning assignments translate the skills and knowledge described in the text into learning objectives, example learning activities, and criteria for evaluating mastery. As organized, the model assignments can be used in structured or self-directed instruction. They can be used by students and their supervisors to help organize internships and practica in home health settings. They can also be used by supervisors for on-the-job or in-service training.

Much of the original thinking that gave rise to the present volume was developed as part of a larger model training project called Geriatric Case Practice run under my direction at George Warren Brown School of Social Work, Washington University in St. Louis, Missouri. These original materials were developed through the combined efforts of the project staff and practicing home health professionals who served on the project's home health advisory panel.

Geriatric Case Practice designates an approach to professional practice with the elderly that emphasizes the psychosocial aspects of care across the continuum of health and social services. Social workers and nurses are most typically the professionals responsible for the social and psychological well-being of elderly patients or clients, although any professional or paraprofessional working with elderly persons in any of the social or health care services that form the continuum may serve the functions. The physical, functional, psychological, and social status of the older person changes over time, necessitating changes in the type of care needed and the range of services required. The outlook presented in **Geriatric Case Practice** views the health care and social services needs of the elderly as a service continuum where home health care serves as one key service along the continuum. Other services along the continuum include case management in the community, acute health care provided in hospitals, chronic long-term care provided in nursing homes, and terminal care for the dying in hospice. To serve the psychosocial needs of the elderly, the practitioner working with the elderly needs an understanding of how each individual service setting operates even if the practitioner works primarily within one setting. Other volumes in the **Geriatric Case Practice Training Series** examine these other service settings. The intent of the training series as originally conceived is to help prepare geriatric workers to take on the role of serving as private practice case managers because such professionals would need to have skills and knowledge across the health care continuum.

The present volume has the distinct honor of being authored by one of the preeminent scholars in the home health care field, Lenard W. Kaye, D.S.W., Professor of Social Work and Associate Dean of the Graduate School of Social Work and Social Research at Bryn Mawr College.

Joel Leon, Ph.D.
Series Editor
Associate Professor & Director of Research
Division for Aging Studies and Services
George Washington University Medical Center

Acknowledgments

The author wishes to acknowledge the support of those who aided immeasurably in the preparation of this book.

First and foremost I offer my heartfelt thanks to my wife, Susan I. Reisman, for contributing her professional perspective on community intervention based on her work in geriatric social work practice.

Appreciation is extended to Joel Leon for first articulating the idea for the **Geriatric Case Practice Training Series** and inviting me to prepare this volume. Marquita Flemming, my editor at Sage Publications, was instrumental in ensuring that this volume be carried to fruition. She is a woman of great patience and wisdom.

I am very grateful to Timothy P. Cousounis and Ann Burack-Weiss for their sharp-eyed reviews of the manuscript. Their recommendations were insightful and reflective of their superb professional skills in gerontological community care.

1

The Practice of Home Health Care

Our discussion of geriatric case practice in home health care builds on the central assumption that home health care is both a field of service in its own right and, at the same time, it is counted among an expanding continuum of interventive strategies for the elderly and disabled experiencing varying degrees of functional incapacity due to mental and/or physical decline. This chapter begins by placing home care services in the larger context of gerontological services and then proceeds to identify the professional roles, sources of stress, knowledge, skills, attitudes, and personal qualities especially attributable to the professional home care case practitioner. It subsequently addresses the range of clients and problems that home care personnel are likely to be working with as well as the range of organizational auspices out of which home health care initiatives emerge. Finally, the merits of utilizing self-evaluation techniques by personnel in home health care will be considered.

Practice in Home Health Care

The Place of Home Care in the Service Continuum

It is important for the case practitioner in home health care to appreciate the fact that services delivered in the home of the older adult or disabled person can vary considerably. No single type of service can be expected to satisfy the exceedingly wide range of needs that the completely or partially homebound person may display.

The continuum of care for the homebound or semihomebound elderly in the community begins, on the lower strata, with small-scale, rather disparate services such as friendly visiting, Meals-on-Wheels, escort service, chore service, "life line" type programs that provide the aged with a mechanical means of communication with service providers (emergency response systems), daily friendly telephone calls, and daily personal checks by the postal service (available in many larger cities).

Mid-range home health care services are those provided by a variety of semiprofessional personnel including home attendants, homemakers, home health aides, and personal care assistants. Traditionally designated ancillary or supplemental services by agencies, these types of services frequently combine to form the central core of the home health care agency's available battery of service supports. The responsibilities of these individuals can range from purely household support functions including meal preparation, shopping, laundry, and cleaning to personal care "hands-on" functions such as assistance with grooming, dressing, toileting, and eating to social-therapeutic forms of help such as supportive companionship.

Finally, at the upper end, home health care entails the delivery of an expanding array of more traditional professional service functions including, most frequently, visiting nurse services and home visits by local social workers and, less frequently, periodic assistance from recreational therapists, occupational therapists, physical therapists, dentists, physicians, psychiatrists, speech and language pathologists, nutritionists, psychologists, legal specialists, and clergy.

In reality, as the case practitioner quickly learns, the services outlined above and summarized in Figure 1.1, are more often than not sewn together in patchwork fashion to produce a more or less comprehensive service package encompassing the resources of more than any one community agency can bring to bear. Most often the missing ingredient is that of case management or service coordination—a function that will be referred to throughout this book as an essential responsibility of the concerned case practitioner in home health care. (A more detailed discussion of the use of case management skills during service delivery is found in Chapter 8.) In those communities where the case management function is bypassed,

1. Housekeeping services
   a. Cleaning
   b. Laundry
   c. Cooking/Meal preparation
   d. Shopping
2. Escort services
3. Personal care services
   a. Assistance with bathing
   b. Assistance with grooming
   c. Assistance with eating
   d. Assistance with dressing
   e. Assistance with ambulation
4. Informational and referral services
5. Education, teaching, and training services
   a. Money management
   b. Home management
   c. Nutrition/Diet management
6. Social-therapeutic services
   a. Supportive companionship
   b. Friendly visiting
   c. Telephone reassurance
   d. Personal and family counseling
   e. Needs assessment
   f. Case management
   g. Case termination procedures
7. Nursing/Medically related services
   a. Reinforcing and changing dressing
   b. Maintaining respiratory equipment
   c. Irrigating catheters
   d. Changing colostomy bags
   e. Maintaining medication routines
8. Rehabilitative services
   a. Assistance with exercise routines

Figure 1.1. A Classification of Home Care Functions

home health care services appear to be particularly piecemeal, the result being a vastly lessening level of effectiveness and efficiency during service delivery. Efforts to provide or help access needed services can greatly improve the comprehensiveness and continuity of care to the older adult, as demonstrated in this scenario:

During your routine home visit to Mrs. Palmer you notice a number of bruises and scratches on her arms and face. You question your client regarding the origin of the injuries and are informed that they were inflicted by her daughter during a recent visit. Mrs. Palmer confides that her daughter has had psychiatric problems for several years and has been physically abusive in the past. Your client wants desperately to help her daughter, but doesn't know how to do so and, in addition, fears the possibility of continued abuse. Respecting Mrs. Palmer's right to confidentiality, you ask her permission to contact the local victim services organization to help her protect herself and deal with her familial situation. In addition, you furnish her with information on a community mental health program for her daughter, should she choose to assist her daughter in seeking help. In this situation knowledge of available services was an asset to the case practitioner attempting to provide comprehensive care.

Home health care, by definition, assumes a more sophisticated repertoire of services being offered than any single intervention described above. Because home health is more often than not tantamount to the delivery of a service package, case management becomes a particularly essential ingredient.

At this time probably the most sophisticated and comprehensive form of home health care available is long-term health care. Long-term home health care programs offer, in addition to a home health aide or home attendant, regular nursing service, social service, Meals-on-Wheels, and, when necessary, the provisions of physical therapists, all as part of the basic service package. Naturally the case management role is explicit under such circumstances and often includes the overseeing of services other than those provided by the home health care agency itself. Information and referral are also standard components of long-term home health care as evidenced by their common role in helping the client in need of more comprehensive or medically related care through eventual nursing home or related institutional placement.

It is important for the case practitioner to remember that home health care services and its myriad of components not only comprise a continuum of services delivered in the older person's home but also represent but a single field of service within the rapidly expanding gerontological services continuum. Tobin and Toseland (1985) offer a classification of these services that differentiates between those that are: (a) community based, (b) home based, and (c) congregate residential and institutional based. They further differentiate between services within each of these three categories, which are geared to meet the needs of the minimally, moderately, and severely impaired (see Figure 1.2). For instance, home repair services are classified as

Degree of Impairment	Community-Based	Home-Based	Congregate Residential and Institutional-Based
Minimal	Adult Education Senior Centers Voluntary Organizations Congegate Dining Programs Individual and Family Information and Referral, Advice, and Counseling	Home Repair Services Home Equity Conversion Share-a-Home Transportation Telephone Reassurance	Retirement Communities Senior Housing Congregate Residential Housing With Meals
Moderate	Multipurpose Senior Centers Community Mental Health Centers Outpatient Health Services Case Management Systems (Social/ Health Maintenance Organizations, etc.)	Foster Family Care Homemaker Meals-on-Wheels Case Management for Family Caregivers and Elderly Impaired Members	Group Homes Sheltered Residential Facilities Board and Care (Domiciliary Care) Facilities Respite Care
Severe	Medical Day Care Psychiatric Day Care Alzeheimer Family Groups	Home Health Care Protective Services Hospital Care at Home	Acute Hospitals Intermediate (Health Related) Nursing Facilities Skilled Nursing Facilities Hospice Care in a Facility

Figure 1.2. A Classification of Services for Older Persons (Focus of Service Delivery)
SOURCE: Tobin and Toseland (1985)

home-based services for the minimally impaired, whereas hospital care at home serves the needs of the severely impaired older adult. Homemaker and Meals-on-Wheels programs are presumed to serve the moderately impaired elderly in their own home.

Because services for the elderly in most communities have not been constructed based on a master plan for satisfying the needs of older adults, the case practitioner is obliged to be an informed provider of care, understanding which services in the community are discrete and which have integrative ties to other programs. The dominating feature of elder care is the discrete model of service rather than the integrated model. As a result the case practitioner's responsibility in performing the service management function is all the more critical.

The practitioner who has assumed the responsibility of maintaining accurate resource files of what services (home based, community based, and congregate or institutional based) are available in a particular community (and which are not) is far more likely to be able to successfully address the changing needs of his or her homebound clients. A convenient source of this information in many large cities is the directory of social and health agencies produced by the local community council or United Way organization. These sources of information on the service network include the local Area Agency on Aging (each county in the United States has one), Social Security and Medicaid offices in the community, and local senior citizen centers.

The case practitioner's *service resource files* need to be updated regularly paying particular attention to:

1. changing eligibility criteria for different services (including age, household composition, availability of other supports, financial status, and functional status requirements);
2. the discontinuation of particular types of services;
3. the initiation of new programs in the neighborhood;
4. the geographic catchment boundaries of programs;
5. the type and range of services offered by programs;
6. the usual waiting periods before service can be provided; and
7. key contact persons with whom application is made.

It is a good idea to think of maintaining gerontological services resource information using computer facilities. Computerized data bases are quickly becoming standard approaches to information maintenance in community agencies. They save space and can be easily accessed and efficiently updated as program information changes. A wide variety of data base management software programs is now available that can fulfill this function in the home health care agency.

Professional Roles

The case practitioner in home health care can be expected to assume an unusually wide range of roles in order to ensure the provision of quality service. Both affective or psychologically supportive roles and instrumental functions are assumed during the average day in home health care. These two dimensions of professional service cross disciplinary lines. That is, regardless of whether case practitioners have been trained as nurses, social workers, occupational therapists, or public health workers, their interventive repertoire will likely entail both dimensions of service delivery (i.e., talk-oriented and physical, "hands-on" care).

Of course, depending on the particular disciplinary background of the case practitioner, a particular set of professional roles will be stressed. Thus nurse practitioners in home health care may emphasize the performance of such concrete tasks as: (a) changing dressings, (b) colostomy care, (c) inserting Foley catheters, (d) monitoring vital signs, (e) health teaching, (f) inserting nasogastric tubes, and (g) monitoring cardiopulmonary status (Ryan & Wassenberg, 1980; Spiegel, 1983; see also Stuart-Siddall, 1986, for an in-depth discussion of the role of the nurse clinician and administrator in home health care).

On the other hand, social work case practitioners will be likely candidates for assuming such roles as: (a) providing casework services, (b) providing program coordination and supervision, (c) providing counseling and advocacy services, and (d) carrying out administrative responsibilities in planning and program development (Axelrod, 1978).

In addition to the skills that are unique to the various disciplines, a common set of universal multidisciplinary case practitioner roles can be identified (Friedman & Kaye, 1979; Kaye, 1985a). They include:

1. *Client-Worker Matching*. The practitioner is responsible for developing a mutually agreeable work plan that should include a process of matching clients and home care personnel such that gender, cultural background, personality, and the like are considered in the assignment process.

2. *Care Plan Preparation*. The practitioner should engage in a planful process that ensures that the elderly client and all involved family supports understand the reasoning behind the fashioning of a particular care plan.

3. *Social Network Integration*. The case practitioner needs to be cognizant of the importance of weaving into the home care plan the

assistance of the client's social supports. This is to be carried out at a realistic and mutually acceptable level of participation.

4. *Provision of Sociotherapeutic Services.* Providing social therapeutic services to families on an as-needed basis is a critical role that affords clients and significant others the opportunity to explore feelings, contribute constructively to the home care plan of service, and remain connected to one another during the course of service delivery.

5. *Client Screening.* The importance of identifying elderly clients with special counseling or protective service needs cannot be emphasized enough. The practitioner assumes the role of client screener whenever possible prior to service initiation so that the case plan and case management functions accurately reflect special client needs.

6. *Resolving Relationship Conflicts.* A process of assessing client expectations and working toward the early resolution of conflict, anger, confusion, hostility, and confusion surrounding the home care relationship is a practitioner responsibility that can pave the way to a mutually agreeable service delivery sequence.

7. *Systems Linkaging.* The role of the systems linkage specialist is one that relates directly to the provision of case management services. The practitioner needs to be able to assess when and in what ways the client could benefit from being connected to the larger social, educational, and health care network available in a particular community.

8. *Care Modality Transition Assistance.* Frequently practitioners assume the role of *modality transition specialists.* In these cases they engage in a process of assisting clients and their families as they move through the stages of terminating receipt of home care (or a particular category of home care) and commencing with the receipt of an alternative service package.

In assuming the explicit functions outlined above, the case practitioner ultimately seeks to maximize the elderly person's sense of self-determination and independence in the context of necessarily acknowledging some loss of personal autonomy. Implicit in the case practitioner's stance is a commitment to: (a) engendering a relationship with the client, (b) building upon existing client strengths, (c) advocating on behalf of the client, (d) identifying and analyzing problems, (e) proposing alternative solutions to problems, (f) assisting in identifying the optimal course of action, and (g) personally delivering or ensuring that the needed service is provided by others.

Foregoing any one role responsibility can have disastrous effects. For example, failure of program staff to adequately prepare all significant parties (i.e., to mutually contract with client and family) may lead to grossly inaccurate perceptions of service (Friedman & Kaye, 1979; Kaye, 1985a):

1. Clients may expect home care personnel to perform a certain set of functions that are very different from those included in the worker's job description.
2. Clients may expect home care personnel to provide companionship after normal working hours.
3. Clients may harbor unrealistic standards with regard to the performance of home care staff.
4. Clients may expect home care personnel to be similar to themselves in race, religion, cultural preference, age, and personal preferences.
5. Families of clients may be confused about their role in the home care service plan.

The absence of mutual understanding in the process of developing a contract with the potential client and significant others can lead to otherwise avoidable problems as indicated in the following vignette:

Eight weeks ago Mrs. Henry was referred to your agency by her son, who stated he was no longer able to provide needed care to his mother in his home and was therefore requesting home care services. You now receive an unexpected telephone call from her angry son who criticizes you for not doing your job. Upon further investigation, it is discovered that the son's main motive in referring his mother to your agency was to access counseling services for his mother to improve her relationship with him. Because his input was not sought in the contracting phase and he was not made fully aware of the limitations of service, he held unrealistic expectations that led to dissatisfaction and confrontation with the case practitioner.

It should have become clear by this point that considerable role flexibility is a common occupational hazard for the home health care case practitioner. The case practitioner does not, as a rule, have the luxury of maintaining a single specialized role during all phases of service planning and delivery. Instead, the successful professional will maintain a healthy sense of flexibility in terms of the range of functions he or she is ready and willing to fulfill. True, limits must be drawn defining what is appropriate and what is inappropriate behavior, but frequently, effective and responsive practice hinges on a good measure of liberal thinking in this regard. Be aware, however, that policies regarding role boundaries vary from agency to agency and that personal liability issues may come into play when boundaries are not respected.

Service Delivery Stress and Burnout

A significant danger in the field of home health care has tended to be personnel overload or burnout resulting in part from the continued accrual of both physical and emotional stress and strain associated with the job. Of course the "burnout syndrome" is not unique to home health care nor to employment in work with the aged. Yet staff turnover seems to be a particularly disturbing and disruptive occurrence in services to the aged and disabled in their homes, and its manifestation can have direct consequences for the well-being of service recipients.

Various factors have been identified as contributing to personnel turnover in home care. Sources of stress among semiprofessional staff (e.g., homemakers, home attendants, chore workers, etc.) can include:

- A lack of gratification due to either the inability of the infirm elderly to recognize/acknowledge staff effort or due to a lack of respect for such work by the general public
- Low salaries and poor fringe benefit packages for many workers
- Little opportunity for upward mobility or career advancement
- The physically demanding nature of the work
- The extended periods of isolation experienced by the worker who is restricted to the client's apartment
- Frequent ethnic, racial, and cultural differences between client and paraprofessional that can lead to misunderstandings, frustration, and even hostility during the course of service delivery
- Often the absence of adequate supervisory mechanisms provided by the home care agency

Sources of stress for professional case practitioners and equivalent personnel in home health care can include:

- Demanding caseloads in both number and difficulty
- The inability to maintain a firm grasp of the supervisory and monitoring function due to the extent of geographic isolation inherent in this field of service
- The demands of continuous travel in what can be unsafe and threatening neighborhoods
- The demands surrounding the supervision of paraprofessional staff, many of whom are experiencing a similar set of personnel strains in the workplace
- Low salaries as compared to peers in other settings
- Excessive paperwork, especially in those agencies that are recipients of public reimbursement for services rendered
- The demands associated with the stressful, emotionally-laden atmosphere of the client's home environment (Kaye, 1985a; Kaye & Reisman, 1991b)
- The fact that home care services are considered ancillary services of low priority and workers occupying such positions are perceived to be of low status within the human services field (Kaye, 1982; Kaye, 1985a; Kaye & Reisman, 1991b)
- The difficulties associated with repeated confrontations with disease, illness, death, and dying among clients and consequent confrontations with one's own mortality and personal finitude (Monk, 1981)

The two sets of personnel stress factors presented above are not mutually exclusive. Paraprofessional and professional staff in home care frequently have a subset of mutual concerns that must be grappled with on a daily basis at work. To acknowledge the commonality of stress with colleagues at various levels in the home care organization can often help in reducing the sense of individual responsibility one thinks he or she needs to assume in dealing with the frustrations common to this service sector.

Given the fact that home care staff are frequently beset by demands from every conceivable direction, what actions can be taken to lessen the deleterious effects? A range of actions is recommended that stress the importance of: (a) handling personal reactions while on the job, (b) organizing one's workload, and (c) taking an activist stance on home care issues.

A Course of Action in Addressing Worker Overload

1. Keep a careful eye open to the telltale signs of worker stress in yourself and in your staff. Increased occurrences of conflict, hostility, depression, and apathy are frequent expressions of stress buildup.

2. Take action when the evidence has presented itself. Confront the issue in supervisory sessions, exploring possible strategies to reduce the cause of stress through alterations in staff assignments, schedules, or responsibilities, changes in agency policy, or by means of the act of ventilation itself.

3. Participate in staff support groups in your agency or with staff from other agencies so that similar concerns and issues can be identified and grappled with. Simply recognizing that your problems are not unique can serve to lessen some of the frustration. Networking and mutual aid initiatives work.

4. Allocate your time judiciously. Limitations need to be set in terms of the amount of time and self you are able to give to any one client. Draining your reservoir of emotional and physical energies on a single client does not serve a positive function in the long run either for your clients or for yourself. Effective time management is key here.

5. Be organized in performing your case load tasks. Silverstone and Burack-Weiss (1983b) recommend dividing tasks into three general categories: a) tasks related to the case plan, b) paperwork tasks required by your agency and/or regulatory body, and c) tasks requested by clients, family members, and staff that are unrelated to the case plan. They recommend partializing and prioritizing these responsibilities, apportioning a certain amount of your day to each set of tasks.

6. Take full advantage of opportunities in continuing education, in-service training, and attendance at community conferences and workshops. Updating skills on a regular basis is self-reinforcing and provides for a healthy professional orientation to your field of service. Remember, home health care is a burgeoning area of practice with new technologies and methods being developed at an extremely rapid pace.

7. Identify with professional associations, local organizations, and advocacy groups in community-based care. Organizations such as the National HomeCaring Council, the National Association for Home Care, the National Council on the Aging, the Gerontological Society of America, and the American Society on Aging regularly organize special programs on topics in community-based care and provide a forum for case practitioners to disseminate information about their experiences in the field.

8. Advocate for policy changes both within your own agency and in the field of home care generally. Present testimony, attend public hearings, and participate in policy and social action committees in your community using your experience and those of your colleagues as evidence for promoting changes in the field.

9. Finally, accept the reality of turnover in home health care. Services that are evolving must expect some degree of ongoing flux in terms of staffing patterns. Plan accordingly, maintaining backup contingency plans that can be put into action to shore up gaps as they arise in your program.

Home Health Care Practice

Knowledge, Skills, and Attitudes

The successful practice of home health care requires the thorough blending of relevant information, effective method, and enlightened values and personal orientation to service delivery. This special mix of knowledge, skills, and attitudes should reflect several basic beliefs espoused by the home health care professional:

1. A steadfast commitment to maximizing the capacity for independent functioning on the part of the impaired older adult
2. A genuine concern for satisfying the needs of the older person who is experiencing decline, whether it be permanent or temporary, in his or her physical and/or mental capacities
3. A firm confidence that home health care has the capacity to delay and/or prevent institutionalization of the older person
4. An unfaltering willingness to safeguard the health and safety of home care clients through adherence to established standards of care

It is important to note that these principles of orientation to home care assume the equal importance of knowledge and compassion in meeting client objectives in home care. Flexibility, empathy, and decision-making capacity combine to create the effective staff person.

Family-like qualities in the home care worker have proven to be of distinctive importance during service delivery. A study by Kaye (1982) found that both paraprofessional and professional workers in home care assigned major importance to familial or affective orientations to service provision. The significance of such qualities as sensitivity, caring, and warmth cannot be overstated. Such qualities far outweighed more traditional instrumental qualities such as worker discipline and logic. On the other hand, the organized, efficient, and reasonable worker was also accorded high marks in describing the qualities of successful home care personnel. Clearly, a mix of personal and workplace qualities or attitudes is crucial.

In general, the skills that are unique to the various health and social service professions (e.g., nursing, social work, medicine, psychology, recreational therapy, psychiatry, occupational and physical therapy, speech and language therapy, etc.) are applicable to home health care with several major exceptions. The exceptions to the rule derive from the special nature of this field of service.

Home care is unique in that service takes place in the personal confines of the client's home. No other service intervention can make such a claim. And herein lies the rub. Professionals who ultimately assume the responsibilities of case practitioners and similar such titles in home care, have, almost invariably, been trained to deliver service in either institutional or agency settings. Working in the home requires a very different perspective—one that is especially sensitive to the delicate "host-guest" relationship that inevitably evolves as service commences. Home health care personnel need to be sensitive to the psychological and emotional implications for the older person of having to receive help with the basic tasks of daily living in their own apartments and private houses—tasks that were performed in the past with little time and effort. Invasion of privacy issues, loss of control and autonomy, pressures toward compliance, depression, fear of death and dying, all can surface in any given case. The simple reality that meals may no longer be prepared in the precise personal way they were in the past can set off a major emotional outburst between client and worker.

The tasks of supervision are especially affected by the special characteristics of the home environment. Case practitioners with supervisory responsibilities will have to devise a special set of strategies that will overcome the difficulties of monitoring services and performing quality control functions of home-delivered care. Individualized and group supervisory methods will need to be combined with team approaches as well as extensive use of nontraditional supervisory methods including periodic on-site visits and use of telephone exchanges. Respecting the client's home setting while enhancing the therapeutic aspects of that setting are central to the supervisory process as is compensating for the physical distance of the home from the agency's back-up resources. Frequent changes in those personnel assigned caregiving responsibility in the home also serve to complicate the supervisory process (National HomeCaring Council, 1982). The benefits of self-evaluation should also be recognized. (See the final section of this chapter for a discussion of self-evaluation techniques.) Of course the good supervisor will also possess excellent verbal and written communication skills, problem-solving expertise, leadership capacity, and, particularly important in this field, the ability to motivate and maintain the enthusiasm of his or her supervisees.

Professionals and paraprofessionals will therefore need special training in the adaptation of their specialized skills to home-delivered care (National HomeCaring Council, 1982). Because formal professional academic programs rarely provide skills-development preparation in the context of the home, the worker is obliged to take full advantage of ongoing staff development and training programs as they arise. This will be especially important as new practice techniques and equipment for home maintenance become more widely available.

In addition to the "home-tailored" skills unique to the various disciplines involved in home care case practice, there are certain basic skills needed for which special training is desirable. These include:

- Knowledge of the aging process and sensitivity to the impact of disability, dependency, and loss of privacy on the home care client
- Appreciation of the merits of the team approach to home care in addressing the multiple needs of the homebound
- Observational and diagnostic capacity for identifying change in client symptomatology and needs

- Appreciation for maintaining the integrity and viability of the client's natural helping network by means of supplementation rather than substitution. (This includes an understanding of family dynamics and the capacity to work with the family unit.)
- Ability to withstand strain and to respond flexibly to client demands
- Skill at navigating the bureaucratic tangle of health and social entitlements and services available to the elderly in the community

Range of Clients and Problems

The range of potential home health care service recipients is exceedingly large and diverse. It encompasses: (a) the developmentally disabled, (b) post-hospitalization patients, (c) the disabled and chronically impaired of all ages, (d) the mentally ill, (e) the terminally ill requiring hospice care at home, (f) newborn infants and their mothers, and (g) abused older adults and children.

While this book emphasizes services for older persons, the fastest-growing segment of the population, home health care has had a long tradition of responding to the needs of individuals of all ages. Indeed, many of the skills considered essential in this book for successful services delivered to the aged are transferable to younger client groups in need of home-based care. (See Ahmann, 1986, for a comprehensive guide to providing home care for the high-risk infant or Gilbertson, 1981, for a guide to providing homemaker-home health aide services for the person with developmental disabilities.) Many would argue, however, that the aged, by virtue of the extended period of time in which they have lived, represent a particularly heterogeneous group, presenting the case practitioner with a seemingly endless variety of needs and requests for support. It is this diversity in the older population that speaks to the importance of establishing a wide range of flexibly applied interventive strategies in the home situation.

There are numerous situations of both a personal and environmental nature that can necessitate the initiation of home care services for the older adult. The presence of one or more of these risk factors dramatically increases the likelihood that home care will be needed. Case practitioners involved in the referral process need to maintain an especially keen eye on elders in the community who display any of the following risk factors:

1. *Acute Disability.* Unexpected accidents such as falls and acute illness can signal the need for time-limited home care assistance. Service will likely be needed only as long as the healing process is underway or recovery progresses.

2. *Chronic Disability.* Long-term impairment due to a chronic illness or disease (e.g., stroke, heart disease, arthritis) is an all too common factor instigating the need for service. Frequently service is needed for an extended period of time in such cases.

3. *Absence or Lack of Social Supports.* While the majority of community care for the elderly continues to be provided by the family unit, it is not unusual for individuals who live into their seventies and eighties to outlive a large segment of their natural support network comprising family, friends, and neighbors. If significant others have not been outlived, they may have their own problems with which to grapple, leaving them unavailable to care for others. Weak or nonexistent support networks place the impaired older person in severe jeopardy.

4. *Diminished Ability to Handle ADL.* The functional and physical activities of daily living must be performed if an individual is to continue living with any degree of dignity in the community. The inability to accomplish one or more of these basic tasks is a prime measure of need for outside assistance.

5. *Psychological or Cognitive Decline.* Periods of mental confusion or disorientation place the older adult residing in the community at high risk. Such an individual may be a danger both to himself and others. Home care can serve as an effective intervention when the condition is episodic and intermittent assistance is adequate.

6. *The Experience of a Traumatic Event.* It is not unusual for a sudden, highly distressful event to exacerbate potentially impairing conditions in the elderly. The death of a spouse, sudden alterations in the environment, temporary or permanent loss of autonomy, relocation of a close friend, a robbery or mugging, all can bring on a downturn in physical or mental health and the need for outside help.

Depending on the nature of the precipitating factor, home health care can assume remedial/rehabilitative, custodial/maintenance, or some combination of these two categories of functions. It is important not to assume that it will necessarily fulfill one or the other function but, rather, to judge each case individually, based on the presenting problem(s).

Home Health Auspice

Home health care services are provided by any number of organizational sources, including public programs, vendor programs, private/non-for-profit groups, and proprietary or for-profit organizations. Similarly, home care services may be freestanding, which is the exclusive program offered by an agency, or it may be one of many services offered by a facility or company.

More and more hospitals and long-term care facilities are offering home care services, which means that health-related and skilled nursing care, hospital services, and apartments for the well aged may comprise the total service package. Similarly, an increasing number of national home health care companies now offer not only personnel-based services, but are in the business of selling and renting durable medical equipment and health products as well. Home care services may be relatively small ancillary programs attached to large organizations (e.g., a home health care program housed within a large-scale urban hospital and medical center). In the case of private auspice home care programs, services are frequently third-party reimbursable by Medicare, Medicaid, private insurance policies, Blue Cross-Blue Shield, Health Maintenance Organizations (HMOs), and group health plans.

The point to remember is that the nature of agency auspice, in large part, determines: (a) the type of financing mechanisms available to the agency and its clientele, (b) the extent to which a social or medical emphasis dominates the service philosophy, (c) the type of personnel who are likely to be employed, (d) the range of services offered, (e) the criteria for participation, and (f) the characteristics of the client population.

The professional case practitioner should not assume that these factors will remain constant from one agency to the next. In fact, the home care agency network is well-known for rather dramatic fluctuations in eligibility criteria, services offered, and so on. The professional who stays informed of these differences from one agency to the next will be better able to make appropriate and timely referrals for his or her elderly clients.

The Role of Self-Evaluation

Because of the special nature of home health care practice, which is performed primarily in the older person's home and, therefore, out of sight of other members of the traditional home care team as well as supervisory staff, it is crucial that personnel in this field engage in a regular process of ongoing self-evaluation of performance. The difficulties inherent in maintaining effective peer and supervisory review procedures in home care make self-assessment particularly crucial. Of equal importance is establishing an organization environment that encourages and rewards honest self-reporting to superiors as well as requests for direction and advice regarding practice. Case practitioners should advocate for this kind of open-door atmosphere in their agencies, especially for those staff engaged in the most intensive and continuous periods of direct service (e.g., homemakers, home health aides, home attendants, chore workers, etc.). Self-assessment will fail miserably if an atmosphere of distrust and fear of criteria exists in the agency.

A formal mechanism whereby home care personnel are obliged to follow a regular schedule of self-evaluative procedures is recommended. While each agency will want to tailor its self-evaluation tools to meet its particular needs, a series of basic questions seem apparent. The self-assessment should entail attention to the following questions concerning personnel performance:

1. To what extent are those services stipulated in the case plan being delivered?
2. Are services being delivered in a timely fashion? Are they being delivered safely?
3. What aspects of home care have you found to be the most demanding? What issues most frequently require supervisory consultation?
4. What aspects of the care plan do you feel able to perform most effectively? Which dimensions of care do you feel less effective in performing?
5. What kinds of client problems do you feel most confident in addressing? Which do you feel less confident in addressing?

6. Are you satisfied with the quality of the working relationship you have established with your client? With other members of the client's support system?

7. How well do you interact with other members of the home care team? Do you feel you relate more or less effectively with those staff having similar responsibilities as yourself as compared to those with different kinds of functional responsibilities?

8. In what areas of home care practice do you feel you could benefit from more skills training? What areas of your work could improve with increased on-the-job experience?

9. How would you rate yourself in terms of the following home care worker qualities? ____disciplined ____sensitive ____logical ____warm ____organized ____caring ____reasonable ____efficient ____friendly ____responsible

10. To what extent do you find you are able to communicate effectively, both orally and in writing, with your clients? With other staff? With other agencies in the community service network?

11. To what extent do you feel you comply with your home health care agency's policies and procedures?

2

The Policy Context

This chapter addresses a series of macro issues in home health care. That is, the larger context in which home-delivered services are provided will be considered with special attention directed at agency, state, and federal policies that influence the case practitioner's experience. Funding source requirements, community resources, and agency regulations will all be considered. Documentation skills for home health care practice will be reviewed as well.

Influence of Policies on Practice

Policy Issues and Service Coverage

Two levels of policy have a distinct effect on the organization and practice of home health care: governmental and agency based. Governmental policies impact on practice in two major ways: (a) through the promulgation of regulations surrounding home care program funding and third-party payments, and (b) through laws regulating home care program organization. The home health care case practitioner can benefit from an awareness of both types of policies. The case practitioner who performs managerial and administrative functions in combination with case practice functions has a responsibility to be particularly well versed in such matters.

Sources of funding for home health care emerge from at least five federal programs. Medically oriented home care tends to be funded through Titles XVIII and XIX of the Social Security Act. On the other hand, programs that emphasize social and personal care services are supported through Title XX of the Social Security Act and Title III of the Older Americans Act. In addition, the Veterans Administration provides funding for both social and health-related home care services. (Of course, a substantial portion of home care is financed through private and commercial insurance companies, charitable and philanthropic groups, and out-of-pocket expenditures by the elderly themselves and their families.)

The task of the case practitioner in keeping abreast of regulatory policy in terms of governmental reimbursement for home care services is a particularly difficult one. This is due to the fact that reimbursement policy varies considerably from one funding source to the next. Variation is to be found in types of services covered, funding levels, service duration limitations, service eligibility rules, target group emphases, and the extent to which available funds are actually utilized (Kaye, 1985a). Added to this is the fact that regulatory policy is not constant. Changes in regulatory criteria are occurring at a rapid pace combined with periodic fluctuations in the manner in which eligibility for coverage is being interpreted. Figure 2.1 summarizes the major differences in coverage of the four major legislative mechanisms financing home care services for the aged and disabled.

Third-party payments (e.g., a client being covered by Medicaid or Medicare for services received) are determined by a variety of factors, including client diagnoses, the types of services that are required, the category of personnel providing care, and the circumstances under which assistance is offered (e.g., hours of services offered per day or week). Certain services and periods of coverage are not reimbursable. Furthermore, certain agencies may not be reimbursable under Medicaid or Medicare because they are uncertified.

What follows is a review of the types of coverage available through the major legislative mechanisms mandating home health care.

Medicare: Title XVIII of the Social Security Act

Medicare coverage of home health care is authorized by sections 1812, 1832, and 1835 of Title XVIII of the Social Security Act. Either

Policy Criterion	Legislative Mechanism			
	Title XVIII (SSA)	Title XIX (SSA)	Title XX (SSA)	Title III (OAA)
Type of service coverage	Professional/ Paraprofessional	Professional/ Paraprofessional	Paraprofessionals	Paraprofessionals
Service duration	Short term	Short term/Long term	Short term/Long term	Short term
Funding time horizon	Ongoing	Ongoing	Ongoing	Time limited
Extent of service coverage	Part time	Part time	Part time	Part time
Service eligibility	Universal	Selectivistic/Means tested	Selectivistic/Means tested	Universal
Target group	Elderly (65+)	Poor (ADC-SSI)	Poor, low, and middle income	Elderly (65+)
Funding type	Open ended	Open ended	Closed ended	Closed ended
Utilization of provisions	Low	Low	High	High
Quality controls	Federal	Federal/State	State/Local	State/Local

Figure 2.1. Comparisons of Four Legislative Mechanisms Mandating Home Care Services for the Aged and Disabled

Part A (Hospital Insurance) or Part B (Medical Insurance) can pay for service. Eligibility criteria center around the need for intermittent skilled nursing, physical, or speech therapies. Confinement to one's home is required as is physician's certification of need and establishment of the home health care plan. There are no time limitations for coverage (i.e., no limitations on the maximum number of allowable visits) and no requirement for prior hospitalization as long as all conditions for eligibility are satisfied.

Medicare coverage is not available for those clients who are solely in need of custodial or maintenance care, assistance in performing the activities of daily living (e.g., household services, shopping, meal preparation, assistance with bathing, dressing, etc.), or medical social services. These services, as well as use of medical supplies, appliances, and some rehabilitation equipment, however, are fully paid for when the older person is confined at home. Reimbursement of support services in the home centers on personal care provided by a home health aide. Homemaker services are not eligible for coverage unless the client elects hospice coverage. Medicare can continue to pay for home health visits as long as occupational therapy continues to be needed even if skilled nursing, physical, or speech therapies are not.

Funding for Medicare home health services is open ended; that is, there is no cap on the amount that may be expended, but utilization patterns reflect low levels of expenditure. Reimbursable home care services must be provided by a certified home health agency. In local communities Medicare reimburses certified home health agencies in a manner similar to that of hospitals—insurance companies and similar fiscal intermediaries assist in the administration of the program, processing claims, determining eligibility, and reimbursing "reasonable costs."

The case practitioner should be aware that there are periods during which eligibility for coverage may be more or less severely assessed. A climate of hospital cost containment may be combined with an effort to limit reimbursement for community-based services such as home health and hospice services as well. During those periods when the assessment process is strictly performed and regulations are narrowly interpreted, rejection rates increase dramatically. During such times the worker has a particularly strong responsibility for amassing well-documented evidence concerning a client's eligibility. The role of advocate comes into play in no uncertain terms during these times, with the responsibility of the practitioner being one of ensuring that those clients who are eligible for third-party reimbursement actually receive it. Of course, case practitioners and their agencies have to decide during such periods whether or not they will provide a client with a particular service, knowing full well that reimbursement may be denied by the fiscal intermediary such as a Blue Cross plan, another private insurance company, or the federal government itself at a later date.

Case practitioners should also realize that the advent of DRGs (Diagnosis Related Groups) enacted under federal law in 1983 has resulted in an increase demand for home care services due to reduced periods of hospitalization for many individuals. The fact is that the Prospective Payment System (PPS) of Medicare reimbursement has prompted hospitals to discharge patients earlier than they would have in the past (National Health Publishing, 1985). A good number of these patients require follow-up care, and herein lies the critical role that home health care and hospice programs have come to play. Home care personnel can be expected to be particularly taxed as a result of these policy changes.

Figure 2.2 summarizes the range of skilled intermittent services covered by Medicare. Medicare does not cover such services as full-time nursing care at home, drugs and biologicals, home-delivered meals, blood transfusions, and, as mentioned earlier, homemaker services.

Beginning in 1983 Medicare was expanded to include coverage of hospice care in the person's home. Individuals with a terminal illness can receive a comprehensive set of medical and support services including those outlined in Figure 2.2. The mission of hospice care is to provide noncurative care to the terminally ill—only pain-relieving medications and treatments are offered. The underlying philosophy includes the patient's right to death with dignity in the familiar surroundings of family, friends, and cherished possessions. Hospice services may be offered by hospitals, home health care agencies, nursing homes, or community-based organizations. Care must be provided by a Medicare-certified hospice if coverage is to be approved. Covered services include: (a) physician's services; (b) nursing services; (c) medical appliances and supplies (including outpatient drugs for symptom management and pain relief); (d) home health aide and homemaker services; (e) physical, occupational, and

Part-Time Skilled Nursing Care

Foley insertion	Decubitus care
Venipuncture	Bladder instillation
Skilled observation	Postcataract care
Restorative nursing	Teach gastrostomy feeding
Wound care/dressing	Administration of vitamin B-12
Administration of I.V.s	Administer care of trachiotomy
Preparation/Administration of insulin	Teach ostomy or Ilio conduit care
Teach nasogastric feeding	Chest physiogamy
Reinsertion of nasogastric tube feeding	Teach administration of injection
Teach care of trachiotomy	Teach parenteral nutrition
Teach diabetic care	Teach inhalation procedure
Administer inhalation procedure	Bowel/Bladder training
Administer other IM/Subq.	Disimpaction/F.U. enema
Other (as specified under orders)	

Speech Therapy

Transfer training	Passive exercises
Therapeutic exercise	Active exercises
Establishment of maintenance program	Proprioceptive neuromuscular
Evaluation	facilitation
Gait training	Resistive exercises
Chest physiotherapy	Stretching exercises
Whirlpool	Ultrasound
Other (as specified under orders)	Prosthetic training

Occupational Therapy

Evaluation	Activities of Daily Living
Muscle reeducation	(ADL) training
Other (as specified under orders)	

Speech Therapy

Evaluation	Comprehensive
Language processing	Aural rehabilitation
Speech voice retraining	Alaryngeal speech
Other (as specified under orders)	

Medical Social Services

Personal counseling	Psychosocial assessment
Financial assistance	Arrangement for meals
Placement assistance	Other (as specified under orders)

Home Health Care

Combing hair	Meals preparation
Shaving	Grocery shopping
Bed bath (partial & complete)	Washing clothes
Tub/Shower bath	Housekeeping
Catheter care	Exercise supervision
Change bed linen	Transfers to bed/chair
Ambulation assistance	Other (as specified under orders)

Medical supplies
Durable medical equipment

Figure 2.2. Types of Services Covered by Medicare

speech therapies; (f) medical social services; (g) counseling; and (h) short-term, inpatient respite care.

Whereas home health care under Medicare covers an unlimited number of home visits, hospice care extends for two periods of 90 days each and one 30-day extension period plus an optional permanent extension under the specific condition that the patient remains terminally ill. While the 90- and 30-day periods are routinely provided, in order to receive the final extension the hospice patient must be recertified as terminally ill. Part A and Part B of Medicare may be drawn on to reimburse for hospice services. (*Hospice Care*, in the Geriatric Case Practice series, explores the role of the case practitioner in the hospice setting and examines issues, relevant policies, and interventions related to death and dying in considerable depth.)

The practitioner who has specific questions about Medicare coverage of home health and hospice services should contact the local Social Security office in his or her community. Phone numbers are listed under "Social Security Administration" or "U.S. Government." Be aware also that community legal aide services for the elderly in larger urban communities as well as community advocacy groups specializing in providing technical assistance to the service community are often excellent sources of information and advice on eligibility for entitlements. They can be of assistance as well in briefing you on the various procedures for appealing decisions made by intermediaries concerning client eligibility for coverage. These same organizations are a good source for informing you of changes in the rules that implement the provisions of federal entitlements such as Medicare. For example, the Institute on Law and Rights of Older Adults of the Brookdale Center on Aging at Hunter College in New York City serves as an educational and consultative clearinghouse of information for professionals working with the elderly. The federal agency that administers the Medicare (and Medicaid) program is the Health Care Financing Administration (HCFA).

Home care practitioners who fulfill administrative functions are referred to the following sources for detailed information on current Medicare regulations:

1. The *Federal Register*—a daily government publication that publishes HCFA's notices, proposed rules, and final regulations. Of particular importance is HCFA's annual July schedule of limits and

revisions to the wage index for home health agencies, including commentary and public comments.

2. HCFA's *Manual for Medicare Certified Home Health Agencies and Hospices*. This document explains which services are covered and which clients are eligible for service.

3. *Home Health and Hospice Manual: Regulations & Guidelines*. This comprehensive manual prepared by the editorial staff of National Health Publishing (a division of Rynd Communications, Owings Mills, MD) is a one-volume, loose-leaf manual updating service for administrators in home health and hospice care. It keeps abreast of all regulatory changes coming out of HCFA, including regulations on home health agencies, hospices, and durable medical equipment. It includes a series of "how-to" guides that address start-of-care procedures for new patients, all required forms for agency administration, billing procedures, instructions for filling out claims for reimbursement and developing agency procedures and practices, as well as legal commentary on new developments in the field. Periodic updates are issued and can be inserted into the manual.

Medicaid: Title XIX of the Social Security Act

Medicaid, or Title XIX of the Social Security Act, authorizes reimbursement for such services as home nursing care, home health aides, and personal care services. As in the case of Medicare, Medicaid reimbursable personnel must be employed by a certified home health agency and satisfy federally established standards. In almost all cases services are limited to part-time coverage.

Criteria for eligibility include low income (specific income eligibility levels vary from state to state), nursing supervision, physician's authorization for service, and periodic review of the care plan. The older person does not have to have been hospitalized prior to application. While the number of allowable home visits is not limited by federal law, states may impose their own limitations. Similarly, federal law does not require that service recipients be in need of professional nursing or therapy to qualify for supportive personal care, or be homebound, nor do regulations prohibit the provision of household maintenance and assistance with ADL. Individual states, however, differentially authorize such coverage (presumably to hold down the cost of care).

Procedures for Medicaid reimbursement for local services can vary considerably from state to state. They are based on state-established schedules of maximum allowance. As a rule, Title XIX regulations stipulate a 50-50 federal/state match. This can, however, fluctuate based on regional variations in per capita income. For instance, while the federal government pays more than half of all Medicaid costs (about 55% nationally), it may pay as much as 78% (for Mississippi, the state with the lowest per capita income).

Because Medicaid is actually 55 separate programs (each state and United States territory has its own version), home care administrators and practitioners have a particularly demanding task of being well informed of the programmatic regulations in their own state. Individual state plans can be reviewed at local public health, state welfare, social service, or state Medicaid offices. Some states allow the aged, blind, and disabled to apply for benefits through the local Social Security office. Remember that each state has considerable discretion in terms of the establishment of its own eligibility criteria, service and benefit packages, and rates of reimbursement. Federal Medicaid regulations do require that all participating states (Arizona is the only nonparticipant) minimally provide nursing services, home health aide services, and durable medical equipment. On the other hand, it is at the individual state's discretion whether it offers such services as physical, occupational and speech therapies, medical social services, and personal care assistance.

Elder home care recipients may be eligible for both Medicare and Medicaid. In such cases Medicaid pays for Medicare premiums and deductibles. Medicaid can also cover the cost of those portions of medical expenses delivered in the home that are not covered by Medicare but that are included in a particular state's Medicaid program.

Application procedures are based on need and, thus, elder applicants will require the following:

1. Proof of income level (paycheck stubs, bankbooks, other evidence of savings or assets, other evidence of your income and that of relatives who live with you)
2. Personal circumstances (proof of age, unemployment, disability)
3. Proof of U.S. citizenship
4. Proof of disability and need for home care services (medical records, etc.)

In most states persons eligible for the Supplemental Security Income Program (SSI) are automatically eligible for Medicaid. Once again, however, case practitioners will need to check their own state regulations. Figure 2.3 summarizes the relationship between Medicaid and SSI standards for eligibility in U.S. states and territories. Of course these guidelines are subject to change, and case practitioners will need to keep abreast of such changes in their own communities. Similarly, income and resource eligibility criteria for Medicaid vary by state according to family size.

Title III and IV of the Older Americans Act (OAA)

Home care services offered through the Older Americans Act (OAA) are for adults 60 years of age or over. Unlike Medicare and Medicaid, OAA services are based on closed-ended formula grants to individual states and designated sub-state areas. A higher proportion of OAA funds have traditionally been spent for in-home services than is the case for Medicare and Medicaid although absolute expenditure levels are substantially lower in the case of the Older Americans Act.

The OAA program, which is grounded in the intent to provide comprehensive and coordinated services that promote independence, places priority on serving the low-income, isolated, and minority aged. While individually funded OAA programs differ in the range of actual services offered, authorized services within Title III include:

- Homemaker services
- Home health aide services
- Chore services
- Friendly visiting services
- Telephone reassurance services
- Health education, immunization, and screening programs
- Home repairs
- Home-delivered meals
- Access services such as transportation, outreach, and information and referral
- Legal and other counseling services

States and Territories Where Aged, Blind, or Disabled Persons Receiving Cash Benefits From the Supplemental Security Income Program (SSI) Are Automatically Eligible for Medicaid

Alabama	Georgia	Montana	South Carolina
Alaska	Idaho	Nevada	South Dakota
Arizona	Iowa	New Jersey	Tennessee
Arkansas	Kansas	New Mexico	Texas
California	Kentucky	New York	Vermont
Colorado	Louisiana	Northern Mari-	Washington
Delaware	Maine	ana Islands	West Virginia
District of	Maryland	Oregon	Wisconsin
Columbia	Massachusetts	Pennsylvania	Wyoming
Florida	Michigan	Rhode Island	

States and Territories Where Aged, Blind, or Disabled Persons Receiving Cash Benefits From the Supplemental Security Income Program (SSI) Must Meet Stricter Standards for Medicaid Eligibility

Connecticut	New Hampshire
Guam	North Carolina
Hawaii	North Dakota
Illinois	Ohio
Indiana	Oklahoma
Minnesota	Puerto Rico
Mississippi	Utah
Missouri	Virgin Islands
Nebraska	Virginia

Figure 2.3. Comparison of Eligibility for Medicaid and Supplemental Security Income (SSI)

Area Agencies on Aging, which either provide services themselves or contract with community organizations, are mandated to spend 50% of their Title III allocation for in-home, legal, and access services as listed above unless it can be determined that the community has an adequate supply of such services from alternative sources. Local providers are awarded operating funds on an annual basis. Coverage is time-limited.

Some home care practitioners may find themselves associated with research and demonstration projects funded through Title IV of the Older Americans Act (similarly, such projects are periodically funded with Medicare and Medicaid funds by the Health Care Financing Administration). These programs allow for innovative service delivery designs that are especially geared for those frail elderly who would otherwise be institutionalized. They are, however, designed to be of limited duration and, thus, place additional responsibilities on the practitioner to deal with issues of service termination and case transfer.

Title XX of the Social Security Act

Known as the social services amendment of the Social Security Act, Title XX authorizes a wide variety of home-delivered services. Similar to Medicaid in-home services, Title XX, a grant-in-aid program, allows considerable state discretion in terms of the configuration and scope of available services. Title XX authorizes a 75-25 federal/state matching formula for the majority of available services. Services mandated through this act are geared to: (a) achieving economic self-support; (b) promoting self-sufficiency; (c) reducing neglect, abuse, and exploitation; (d) preventing inappropriate institutionalization; and (e) securing institutional care when other forms of care are not appropriate (Spiegel, 1983). Funding through this legislation is closed ended, with ceilings established according to a state's proportion of the nation's population.

Once again it is critical that the case practitioner be well versed in his or her own state's service configuration because some states attempt to provide home-based services for all individuals while others limit eligibility to income-maintenance recipients. Expenditure levels also vary considerably by state as do local reimbursement methods, including the utilization of competitive bidding models as in California, negotiated rates bidding, as well as direct contracting with individuals for services (Trager, 1980). Practitioners who are associated with Title XX home care need also to keep a close eye on the potential for fraudulent, abusive, and exploitative practices. This is a possibility because training guidelines and provider standards are rather underdeveloped (determined by individual states) and reimbursable personnel comprise a wide variety of providers, including agency personnel, relatives, neighbors, and friends.

One or more of the following home-based services must be provided by each state:

1. Homemaker services, including household maintenance care such as meals proportion, laundry, and cleaning
2. Home health aide services, including personal care assistance with the functional activities of daily living (grooming, dressing, eating, bathing)

3. Home management services such as training in meal planning and preparation, budget management, and consumer education
4. Counseling services addressing the social and emotional issues surrounding dependency and health
5. Chore services such as shopping, house cleaning, home repair, yard work, and so on

The provision of homemaker service has traditionally proven to be the most popular in-home service intervention strategy under Title XX.

Other Public and Private Sources of Home Care Funding

Unlike most other sources of funding for home health care, the Veterans Administration provides direct subsidies to the infirm individual's informal supports who provide the elder with day-to-day care in the home. In addition, the Veterans Administration offers the assistance of a multidisciplinary team of professionals who provide posthospitalization care in the home in conjunction with a family member or other informal support who is available to take responsibility for ongoing care. Team members include a physician, nurse, social worker, dietician, and rehabilitation therapist.

Although not consistently available nationwide, federal funding in the form of demonstration grants to existing agencies for Private Sector Sources of Home Care, the expansion of services, and, to a lesser extent, to develop new home health projects has been provided historically by the Department of Health and Human services through its Public Health Service.

Private organizations and providers of third-party payments for homecare are numerous and complex, but hardly comprehensive or well coordinated. They include many longstanding sources and some newer types that have yet to be proven to be good investments for the older person.

Several major health insurance companies have begun to address the problem of personal financing of long-term home care and nursing home care within recent years by offering special policies designed for these purposes or by offering riders to existing policies. Such policies, often experimental in nature, typically cover services required of patients suffering from Alzheimer's disease, osteoporosis, and related infirmities. Reimbursable services covered by these long-term care policies include housekeeping, cooking, shopping, physical therapy, medication administration, and personal assistance while bathing and dressing. Such policies frequently do not require prior hospitalization. Premiums range from $30 to $60 a month or more. Participating companies include Blue Cross, Blue Shield, Metropolitan Life Insurance Company, and the Prudential Insurance Company of America through the American Association of Retired Persons. While desirable in theory, the adequacy of the benefits of such insurance coverage has proven questionable. The case practitioner needs to be aware of certain pitfalls that may befall a client considering long-term care insurance policies. A series of critical questions need guide the professional's assessment of the adequacy of such policies:

1. First and foremost, one must clarify the boundaries of coverage. Is the coverage long-term or limited in duration?
2. Does it cover all types of home care or only specific components?
3. Must the ensured purchase service from only one or a select few agencies?
4. Does the policy *only* cover posthospitalization home care?

In addition, policies that include nursing home benefits tend to demand high premiums, particularly if purchased in the later years of life, and a number of carriers of this type of coverage have gone bankrupt with the exorbitant cost of institutional care. Among the better known programs, Blue Cross-Blue Shield offers a variety of comprehensive plans that cover home care to some extent when specific criteria are met.

A less recognized source of home care coverage is the prepaid group health plan also referred to as HMOs such as Health Insurance Plans (HIP). Many such programs do offer home care benefits as a part of their basic package, while others provide the coverage for a relatively small additional fee. As is the case with other providers, home care entitlements are delivered as a cost-effective alternative to payments for institutional care.

Documentation Skills for Funding Sources

Different funding sources have different expectations in terms of required documentation of services provided. An agency may receive funding from more than one governmental body (e.g., Medicaid at the state level and Medicare at the federal level), each having its own set of documentation requirements. In addition, the agency may be a recipient of funds from a private organization (e.g., the United Way, the Federation of Jewish Philanthropies, Catholic Charities, the Federation of Protestant Welfare Agencies). Monies may be earmarked for specific, discrete program initiatives or may be partially comingled.

In cases of a home care program receiving funding from multiple sources, record keeping can become increasingly time consuming and demanding. Accountability, however burdensome, is crucial. Timely and accurate record keeping better ensures the likelihood of successfully securing ongoing funding.

Funding source requirements aside, quality record keeping often improves the quality of client care. Good documentation practices can promote the delivery of effective and efficient home health care services. Accurate records expedite the monitoring process that is concerned with the quality and ultimate cost of service delivery and care. Brickner (1978) notes that first-rate documentation, including the maintenance of the medical chart, encourages proper patient care through the promotion of communication between personnel during the course of service delivery, at case review sessions, and during supervisory and team conferences. Accurately maintained case records are a critical source of information serving as a physical representation of the client during case planning sessions.

Good documentation practices also serve as a safeguard for the agency in terms of legal and fiscal obligations. Up-to-date records presumably serve to explain, document, and even justify the type and intensity of services delivered. Records should include sign-offs by clients and workers alike authorizing particular types of services at different points in time. Respect for the confidentiality and right to privacy of clients is part and parcel of the process.

Good record keeping also serves to document the scope and breadth of service needs in a particular community. As such, it can serve to justify future efforts at expanding or altering the package of services that a particular agency or network of agencies offers. The advocacy function that can be fulfilled by good program documentation is too often overlooked by agency administrators and case practitioners alike.

Wilson (1980) has identified a series of purposes served by recording of various types in the delivery of social services. Some have been considered in more detail above. All are applicable to home health agency settings. They are:

- Documentation of service activity
- Continuity of service
- Justification of payment from third-party payors
- Quality control
- Statistical reporting
- Supervisory review
- Organizing the worker's thoughts
- Interdisciplinary communication
- Part of an eligibility requirement
- Teaching
- Research
- Agency defense in legal actions
- A therapeutic tool

Among the types of agency protocols that contribute to the documentation base in home health agencies are:

- Patient care screening and intake forms (see Chapter 5)
- Client assessment forms (see Chapter 6)
- Progress report forms
- Medication awareness reports
- Personnel records and worksheets (social service, nursing, medical, home health aide, etc.)
- Medical charts
- Reassessment and evaluation forms (see Chapter 8)
- Discharge and termination sheets (see Chapter 9)
- Periodic agency statistical reports (summaries of clients served, sources and number of referrals, applications accepted, presenting problems, sociodemographic characteristics of clients, type and number of services offered, number of visits made, sources of payment, number and reasons for discharge, numbers and types of referrals made, etc.).
- Quality assurance forms
- Application for reimbursement forms (e.g., Medicaid, Medicare, etc.)

Good sources for examples of documentation maintained by home health programs include *Administrative Policies and Procedures for Home Health Care* (Bulau, 1991), *Clinical Policies and Procedures for Home Health Care* (Bulau, 1986), *High Tech Home Care Plans* (Gould & Wargo, 1987), *Home Health Care—Forms, Checklists & Guidelines* (Aspen Reference Group, 1989), *The Home Care and Documentation Guide: An Orientation and Resource Manual for Home Health Practitioners* (Huebner, 1991).

In order to fully understand the value of good documentation to both client and practitioner, consider the following scenario:

Mrs. Benitez, who has just moved in with her son, is transferred to your home health care agency from another such program in a different state. The admitting case practitioner has had no direct contact with the referring organization; only the written transfer documents are available, and these are found to be incomplete and inadequate. Mrs. Benitez, due to aphasia (impaired ability to use or comprehend words), can provide no information on her case. Her son only knows the client's diagnosis, the medications she must take, and the number of hours of home care received previously. The practitioner has several critical questions that remain unanswered:

- What type(s) of coverage does the client have?
- Are there any dietary restrictions that must be observed?
- Has the client been receiving physical therapy? occupational therapy? speech therapy?
- Have there been episodes of stroke-related aggressive or unpredictable behavior of which the home health care worker should be aware?
- Is the client able to manage any of her ADLs (activities of daily living)?

As a result of poor documentation, the practitioner must make the time and effort to acquire what is available from the referring agency by calling and writing. In addition, the client must be subjected to otherwise unnecessary reevaluation by various members of the multidisciplinary team. Both the client and service provider must pay the price for poor or incomplete documentation.

Technology and Agency Documentation

It is worth pausing to consider the implications of advanced technology for home health care documentation. The technology revolution in the human services is already having a major impact on the organization and delivery of home health services. In turn, it has impacted on the methods by which personnel in this field document service provision. Specialized software is now available that address issues of data management, graphics, word processing, spread-sheets, and telecommunications in the human services. Case prac-titioners can expect to have increasingly frequent contact with com-puterized management information systems that are utilized by home health agencies for budgeting and payroll functions, statisti-cal analyses, scheduling, time sheet generation, case management, and even clinical assessment and diagnostic tasks. An increasing num-ber of computer services are now specializing in serving the home health field.

Case practitioners and other human service professionals will be utilizing innovative computer technology in their daily practice in efforts to automate a wide variety of direct service agency functions. While the practitioner may not be required to possess the skills of a computer programmer, the advantages of direct service providers establishing closer connections to the world of computer technology are increasingly recognized (Kaye, 1991). A survey of clinical soft-ware (McCann, 1987) identified 26 separate microcomputer software programs meant to assist human service providers in performing such functions as psychiatric diagnosis, cognitive rehabilitation, de-cision support, health history and stress inventories, physical and mental health assessments, and health risk appraisals. While elec-tronic data processing technology can assist the practitioner in deliv-ering and documenting clinical service interventions, they are best conceptualized as a supplement rather than a substitute for more traditional comprehensive therapeutic treatment strategies in home health care.

Effective clinical and management documentation procedures in home health require a set of qualities not unlike those in other fields within the health and social services. They include:

1. *Accuracy* in the collection and maintenance of service records
2. *Honesty* in the reporting of events as they transpire during service delivery
3. *Conciseness combined with thoroughness* in the manner in which infor-mation is recorded

4. *Timeliness* in terms of maintaining records that document the changing status of client conditions, clients seen, services provided, hours worked, and so on

5. *Clarity and readability* in the depiction of activities performed and client status so as to render documentation fully transferable from one worker to the next

Community Resources in Home Health Care

It is crucial to have referral data handy in order to avoid the lengthy process of making multiple telephone calls to track down needed services for clients. Development of a "referral resource center" in your agency can provide a system for maintaining up-to-date data once it has been researched. No matter how comprehensive your program may be, there will always be a need for supplemental service supports for your clients. By developing the in-house resource center, you are better informed as to what types of services are available, and you will more easily recognize the appropriate remedies to your client's unmet needs. Furthermore, establishment of the resource center concept informs your program of gaps in service in your community as well. Such knowledge can serve as a springboard to informed program innovation, service expansion, and community advocacy.

Following through on a series of rather simple steps ensures that your resource center will be up-to-date:

1. Collect directories (available from local community boards, community councils, offices on aging)

2. Put your name on mailing lists—Call or write to local agencies serving the aged as well as specialized organizations (i.e., Arthritis Foundation, American Cancer Society, Parkinson's Disease Foundation, Alzheimer's Disease and Related Disorders Association; Area Agencies on Aging, State Offices on Aging)

3. Request brochures and other descriptive literature reflective of gerontological service resources in your community

4. Clip articles from neighborhood and city newspapers that highlight new and innovative programs for older adults in your community or newly discovered treatment techniques for particular illnesses and diseases

5. Make notes to yourself (and systematically file them) each time you discover a new organization or key contact person
6. Compile materials in a resource file that is systematically and logically organized so that information can be quickly retrieved. Categories may include "health care services, victims services, mental health associations, hospice care, respite care," and so on.

The resource file is useful for two purposes: (a) making referrals, and (b) providing information for your continuing care clients. It will be especially helpful if you embark on the resource development project with the cooperation of other staff, thus enabling information to be assembled more efficiently, which will be of relevance to a multidisciplinary group of home health personnel. A secondary benefit derived from this activity is the ongoing personal education of staff.

Sources for Up-to-Date Regulations

The professional case practitioner frequently assumes administrative functions in the home health care agency. As a result, a thorough understanding of regulatory guidelines in the field can be essential. An expanding number of specialized manuals, journals, and newsletters for the community care administrator and program planner have emerged. Several reference sources noted below have been previously discussed in the context of agency documentation.

Specialized Agency Operations Manuals

Aspen Reference Group. (1989). *Home Health Care—Forms, Checklists & Guidelines*. Gaithersburg, MD: Aspen.
Provides practical management materials for home health care administrators including forms and guidelines in the areas of management, human resources, finance, legal issues, marketing, patient care, regulatory compliance, and quality assurance.

Bulau, J. M. (1986). *Clinical Policies and Procedures for Home Health Care*. Rockville, MD: Aspen.
An approach to managing client care with actual clinical policies, procedures, and forms for different categories of client care including client assessment, environment and equipment, safety, medication administration, personal cleanliness, and so on.

Bulau, J. M. (1991). *Administrative Policies and Procedures for Home Health Care* (2nd ed.). Rockville, MD: Aspen.

Provides a compendium of policies, procedures, and forms for various areas of home health care, including general administration, client care, clinical records, education, personnel, quality assurance, and agency services.

Heubner, E. A. (1991). *The Home Care and Documentation Guide: An Orientation and Resource Manual for Home Health Practitioners.* Gaithersburg, MD: Aspen.

Provides guidelines for home health practice including attention to issues of licensure, certification, and accreditation requirements. Sample documents are provided as well as annual updates.

National Health Publishing, Editorial Staff. (1985). *Home Health and Hospice Manual: Regulations and Guidelines.* Owings Mills, MD: National Health Publishing.

A comprehensive listing of Title XVIII (Medicare) regulations governing the administration of home health and hospice agencies and durable medical equipment.

Specialized Journals

Home Health Care Services Quarterly. Laura Reif and Brahna Trager (Eds.), New York: The Haworth Press.

A quarterly professional journal that presents recent research, policy analyses, educational and training curricula, and innovative services delivery in the field of home health care.

Journal of Home Health Care Practice. Jo Ann Parzick and Helen Callahan Triebsch (Eds.), Gaithersburg, MD: Aspen.

A quarterly professional journal that presents practical guidance in the home health field by means of special single topic issues.

PRIDE Institute Journal of Long Term Home Health Care. Ellen R. Harnett (Ed.), New York: PRIDE Institute, St. Vincent's Hospital and Medical Center of New York.

A quarterly publication focusing on policy and service issues in the field of long-term home health care.

Specialized Newsletters

Home Care Economics. R. D. Windley and Helayne O'Keiff (Eds.), Atlanta, GA: American Health Consultants.
A quarterly publication devoted to the business side of home health care including articles, features, and commentary.

Home Health Management Advisor. Kaye Daniels (Ed.), Rockville, MD: Aspen.
A monthly newsletter for home health care managers. Includes management information and advice as well as analysis of management issues facing home health care.

Hospital Home Health. Atlanta, GA: American Health Consultants.
A monthly newsletter for hospital-based home health care programs.

Home Health Line. Karen Rak (Ed.), Port Republic, MD.
A weekly newsletter report on industry and government developments in the field of home health care.

3

The Organizational Context

This chapter directs attention to the organizational structure of home health care. Our attention will be directed to such issues as decision-making perspective, implications for practice of agency chain of command, and fiscal requirements. Finally, the role of the home care professional in the process of program development, design, and evaluation will be explored.

The Organizational Structure of Home Health Care

How Agencies Operate

The term home health agency typically refers to a variety of public and private agencies that participate in the federal health insurance programs of Medicare and Medicaid. These agencies are required to comply with a wide variety of federal, state, and local laws and regulations as well as be certified by a state body designated by the federal government (O'Malley, 1986). Federal Conditions of Participation (Section 1861 of the Social Security Act) must be satisfied to be eligible for reimbursement, and in some states home health agencies are required to obtain a "certificate of need" (CON) before they actually can be state certified and commence operations.

While the home health agency as referred to in this book may also encompass those programs funded through the Older Americans Act, Title XX, and the Veterans Administration, as well as voluntary and freestanding proprietary groups, the organization components remain similar regardless of funding source.

Federal Conditions of Participation require that Medicare and Medicaid-certified agencies have a governing body (the owner or board of directors), an administrator, a supervising physician or registered nurse, and a professional advisory group. Professional nurses have frequently been the individuals predominately involved in home health administration and management (O'Malley, 1986). Even so, social workers, physicians, and public health and administration professionals are also to be found playing dominant roles as home care administrators. Nonparticipating home care programs (those ineligible for Medicare or Medicaid reimbursement) are likely as well to have a governing and/or advisory body as well as a supervising health care professional.

Home care, while not a new idea, has gained substantial popularity only recently. The first organized program is believed to have been that offered by the Boston Dispensary in 1796, although the prototype of today's programs was started at Montifiore Hospital in New York City (Spiegel & Domanowski, 1983; Nassif, 1986-1987). Because of its recent popularity, structural variation in organizational design continues to evolve.

A basic distinction that is currently made is between integrated and freestanding or separate organizations (Spiegel, 1983). Integrated home care programs are lodged within a larger organizational network of services. The most common example is that of hospital-based home care although long-term care institutions such as nursing homes are diversifying into such fields as home health, hospice, and adult day care (Kaye, 1986).

Brickner (1978) has argued that the hospital-based home care program has the greatest likelihood of success given the exceedingly wide range of medical and health-related resources available to serve the homebound older person. He cites the benefits of the hospital's capacity to respond quickly to a medical emergency, provide access to acute care beds, make rapid diagnoses, and benefit from established relations with community agencies and third-party payors. Nevertheless, the debate over a preferential structure continues. Final judgment on the matter is probably premature and, perhaps, irrelevant, given the benefits to be derived from a diversified network of providers.

The adequacy of a particular organizational structure will ultimately be determined by its capacity to sustain continuity in the delivery of services, provide both effective and efficient client care, and maintain a series of fail-safe mechanisms. Fail-safe systems that respond to emergency or unanticipated client need remain one of the major inherent weaknesses in home care today. Traditionally, home care organizational structure has lacked the flexibility, coordination, and necessary resources to react to changing client need. The older adult whose health status suddenly worsens or who loses the services of a family member and is in need of more hours of service or a different range of services is likely to be disappointed in the agency's capacity to respond in a timely fashion. Organization rigidity, promoted by inflexible reimbursement rules and agency regulations, can be the bane of existence for the case practitioner who must ultimately respond to what can be desperate requests for additional aid from the older person.

Staffing in home health care varies with organizational auspice and mandate. Most commonly, home health agencies offer the professional services of physicians, nurses, social workers, and therapists (speech, occupational, physical). Paraprofessional staff may include homemakers, home health aides, home attendants, chore workers, case aides, drivers, and intake workers.

Historically, home care services in the United States have tended to align themselves with the medical model and, in turn, services were provided primarily by professional health services personnel (Ginzberg, Balinsky, & Ostow, 1984). Voluntary visiting nurse services were among the early providers of care serving the subacute elderly population displaying chronic impairment. It was not until the mid-1900s that paraprofessional groups and services appeared, first with homemakers and then home health aides (Mundinger, 1983).

The advent of Medicare altered the structure of home health agencies and the nature of eligibility criteria—the primary change being that agencies were forced to restrict service to clients who displayed an acute care condition, homeboundedness, and the need for skilled care. The medical model continued to prevail under these circumstances. There continues to be a goodly number of home care agencies, however, that place a heavier emphasis on the provision of case management and both social and personal care services.

Other structural variables should, of course, be considered in any discussion of formal agency structure. They include agency auspice (discussed elsewhere), service scope and breadth, division of labor, and target population. Each of these are considered within the context of case practice throughout this volume.

Home Care's Informal Structure

The informal structure of the home care agency is a significant factor defining the nature of practice for the home care case professional. The case practitioner needs to understand the nature of the informal structure because of its inevitable impact on all staff and, ultimately, the client. It is particularly important to distinguish the formal hierarchy that describes the organizational chain of command from the informal "pecking order" in the agency. For this reason it is important in home care, as elsewhere, to establish a rather sophisticated set of political and strategic skills. Similarly, stated policy in home care may differ (sometimes dramatically) from daily practice. The practitioner must consider the potential consequences of abiding by one rather than the other. It would be wise to request supervision should such a conflict arise rather than attempting to grapple with the situation independently.

As an example of strategic use of the informal structure, the following situation describes the steps taken by a case practitioner:

After working for several months as a case practitioner in a large home health care organization, Molly is given responsibility for developing a comprehensive care plan for Ms. Horan. The client's situation necessitates the assistance of a paratransit service to transport her to and from her regular dialysis appointments at the county medical center. Molly is aware that there is a waiting list for the paratransit service and that Ms. Horan's only alternative is to pay for a costly private taxi from her fixed income. She is physically unable to navigate through the barriers of public transportation.

Molly, having come to know the other employees of the agency well, realizes that she has two choices. She can follow the explicit agency procedures dictating reporting relationships and present the case and care plan to her supervisor for review. Her supervisor, fairly new to the agency himself and rather risk-averse in his professional behavior, will advise that Ms. Horan be put on the paratransit waiting list. Molly's other option is first to present the situation to another case practitioner, who, throughout most of her five years with the agency, has been an active member of the local interagency council. This practitioner, Sarah, is very influential at many of the other member agencies, including the paratransit service. Molly is quite sure that Sarah could, at least, get Ms. Horan placed near the top of the waiting list due to the chronic nature of her illness and frequency of treatment.

Recognizing her fellow workers' respective abilities that are unrelated to their formal roles, Molly decides to approach Sarah for assistance before presenting the care plan to her supervisor. The best interests of the client have been considered and there has been no undermining of authority within the organization. In addition, by making the supervisor aware of Sarah's professional contacts in a nonthreatening manner, this informal process can be institutionalized for the benefit of other agency clients.

The Decision-Making Process

One of the most common situations requiring decision making in home care settings is that of determining eligibility for service. Although this is frequently a decision made at the administrative level, the case practitioner may be in a position to have substantial input, especially if that person was involved in the intake process or consulted with regarding the continuation or cancellation of a particular client's plan of care.

Frequently, the three major requirements for home care are homebound status, the need for skilled care, and a physician's written plan for care. As Mundinger (1983) has pointed out, staff are often placed in a position of passing judgment because the first two criteria are open to subjective determination. Among the common dilemmas faced in home care are decisions that need to be made concerning:

1. Choosing between services that will better ensure the client's physical safety (i.e., nursing home care) or their mental/emotional well-being (remaining in their home);
2. Whether clients should be allowed to utilize certain Medicare services even though they may not satisfy all eligibility criteria;
3. Whether clients should continue to receive home care services at the point they no longer satisfy eligibility criteria; and

4. Whether the case practitioner should jeopardize the financial stability of the agency in order that clients receive services for which they are not technically eligible (Mundinger, 1983).

In the latter case the practitioner may be torn between the desire to provide optimal care to all clients and the knowledge that the agency could potentially fail financially and, therefore, leave existing and potential clients without *any* services whatsoever. How does this happen? Take for example a home health care organization in an impoverished rural community. The agency is one of a very few organizations offering health and social services to residents of this underserviced area. Case practitioners, therefore, often have but two choices: (a) provide needed services to clients themselves, or (b) allow clients to go without required assistance. Clearly the former path is the preferable one, but the decision is confounded when some or all of the services are not covered by third-party payments. Thus the agency is, in essence, providing services without compensation. Expenses exceed income in these cases and, without compensating sources of funding, the agency eventually fails financially.

Clearly the four dilemmas cited above are ultimately tied to issues of abiding by informal versus formal structural guidelines (i.e., daily operating procedures versus written policy).

The National HomeCaring Council (1982) has offered a series of guidelines for problem solving in home health care. First, the case practitioner must distinguish between what can be resolved autonomously and what requires supervisory or peer consultation. The following questions should be objectively answered in systematic fashion so that the problem is defined prior to taking action:

1. What is wrong?
2. What are the symptoms or conditions?
3. Where is it located?
4. When did it happen or what time is involved?
5. Who is involved?
6. What are the causes?
7. What can be done?

Ultimately, problem solving will entail a determination of what action is to be taken, by whom, and how. Options should be posed and tested, and the best among them finally selected. The best strategy is that which solves the problem, prevents its reoccurrence, and is practical in terms of time, money, and regulations (National Home-Caring Council, 1982).

It is important that the decision-making process be a collaborative one whereby all staff (and, when appropriate, clients as well) who have a stake in the decision participate in the problem-solving exercise. Final decisions are far more likely to be well conceived and abided by if decisions have been mutually arrived at through staff brainstorming sessions, peer discussion, and interdisciplinary team meetings.

Brody (1977) discusses the decision-making process in the context of making choices concerning whether the older adult should be placed in a long-term care facility or remain in his or her home. Because each client's situation is unique, the question arises time and again without a standardized answer available to the case practitioner. The decision inevitably includes consideration of the following factors: (a) an assessment of the client's physical, functional, and emotional capacity and needs; (b) the client's own personality and inclinations; (c) the client's family situation; and (d) the available resources and informal supports in the client's immediate community.

The goal of decision making is "to determine the best possible plan for the individual older person concerned" (Brody, 1977). The process should, under the best of circumstances, be systematic, continuous, and objective. It is critical to conceptualize the process as an ongoing one—one that is sensitive to changes in client status and need. At the core of care to the frail and vulnerable elderly is the reality of unexpected crisis, medical and social emergencies, and unpredictable requests for assistance. A set of decision-making procedures that is overly regimented is doomed to failure, resulting at the least in insensitive caregiving and potentially as a real threat to the well-being of the client.

Of course one basic factor to be considered is whether the individual meets the criteria for continued home care or nursing home placement. There are many other considerations as noted above, however. Decision making is best conceived as a process and not a solitary act in response to a crisis. Orderly planning includes practitioner assessment of medical, functional, cognitive, social, economic, and personal factors. Increasingly, rather sophisticated client assessment tools are being adopted in home health care to maximize the organized and objective dimensions of the process. (Specific assessment instruments are discussed in Chapter 6.) Remember, however, that preestablished measurement devices merely assist in the decision-making process. When possible, such measures should be supplemented by the contributions of the client, his or her family, and his or her informal support network.

Chain of Command

As indicated earlier, the formal agency structure, in a classical sense, dictates the shape and form of the chain of command. In reality, however, there is generally greater flexibility than is portrayed in the standard agency chart of organization. It is particularly important to be flexible in the home care organization because very often those "on top" of the hierarchy have little or no contact with the client population. In addition, there are frequently several staff who visit the client individually, each with a different professional perspective or orientation, and each receiving a different reaction from and impression of the client. As a result, it is essential that there be a free flow of information and feedback among staff at all levels of the hierarchy.

It is conceivable that the client being served may strongly prefer one agency caregiver among the team providing service. That person may become the most logical and effective staff member to assume responsibility for giving direction to care (National HomeCaring Council, 1982). An open philosophy to designating direction of care can allow for the most effective provision of service to the client. Such a philosophy also ensures that different home care staff will have the opportunity to assume greater responsibility at different points in time—a prerequisite to maintaining worker initiative, motivation, and a sense of professional achievement. Of course such a strategy assumes that those staff members who are granted leadership responsibility display the necessary attitudes, knowledge, and skills that are required for competent performance in this area of practice.

Fiscal Issues

Fiscal audits are a routine part of home care agency operations— both internal (by the agency's own auditors) and by external sources (primarily government and other funding sources). Although non-fiscal staff are rarely involved in such matters, it is crucial that staff be aware that "the records and reports of direct service workers . . . provide the primary source documents for the audit of billing and payroll records" (National HomeCaring Council, 1982). Justification of funds received is attained only when the agency is able to document that it has performed those services for which it claims.

It is also necessary for case practitioners to have a basic understanding of fiscal matters within the organization because it may become necessary to explain to clients and families why services are structured as they are (e.g., due to the need for cost containment and expenditure limitations set by funding sources, certain agencies may be able to provide a lesser number of hours of service each week in particular service categories). By learning about the implications regulations and policies have on funding, case practitioners are able to understand which of the services they provide are reimbursable and which are not. Case practitioners should also have a basic knowledge of costs of various categories of care (e.g., home health versus adult day care versus institutional) in order to assist the client and family in weighing the relative costs and benefits of different levels of available assistance.

Program Development, Design, and Evaluation

Professionals who enter the field of home health care are as likely as any personnel in the human services to perform an exceedingly wide variety of programmatic tasks. Case practitioners will seldom assume responsibility for direct service provision only. Those individuals who enter the field initially as professional frontline personnel seem inevitably to take on indirect service functions somewhere down the road. More likely than not they will eventually perform such functions as supervision, education, and training as well as management and administration. The generic nature of their job responsibilities is due in large part to the small-scale nature of home health care programs, the limited resources that can be earmarked for specialized personnel, and the fact that home health is still in its early evolutionary stages in terms of the degree of functional specificity established within its job classification system.

Among the functions that geriatric professionals in home care frequently come to assume are those of the program development and design specialist as well as the program evaluator. Having had experience as a provider of direct services actually can serve the program designer or evaluator well by informing that person of the specific client needs as well as organizational factors that inevitably impact on the successful development and implementation of home health care programs.

The purpose of this book is not to provide a detailed breakdown of program design and evaluation methodology that can be utilized in home health care. Case practitioners should be aware, however, of the central components of these processes, all of which serve to emphasize the benefits of systematic techniques and methods for conceptualizing and evaluating home health care practice. Home care planning should address a series of classical concerns, all of which aim to give direction in terms of the means or actions by which a program's specified goals will be achieved (York, 1982). Included in the program development process is attention to such matters as:

1. *Problem identification and analysis* (including an assessment of the type and level of need for home care in the community in which programming is to take place);
2. *Program goals and objectives setting* (including the specification of priorities between goals and the development of objectives that are meaningful and realistic for a particular community and home care organization);
3. *Program implementation* (including arriving at the best of alternatives available, establishing program accounting and monitoring mechanisms, budgeting and staffing strategies, scheduling guidelines, etc.); and
4. *Program evaluation* (which is based on the development of measurable criteria, and workable choices for design, data collection, and analysis given the resources available and the requirements for accountability of a given home care agency).

It is quite possible that case practitioners will be asked to participate in selected aspects of program planning. It is not unusual, for example, for home care staff to participate in the performance of a community needs assessment, the results of which are utilized by other staff in planning a new service or modifying an existing one. Similarly, carrying out a program evaluation is frequently considered a specialized task that is performed by particular staff who do not engage in other aspects of agency planning. Just as often, however, external consultants are hired to perform program evaluations. In such cases agency practitioners should still be serving an important role—that of key informant—helping the evaluators design sensitive research instruments that can successfully assess the intricacies of day-to-day programming in the organization.

It is important to remember that there is no single approach to performing home care evaluations. The type of evaluation chosen hinges on a variety of factors including:

- The orientation and expertise of the evaluator
- The interests of the agency
- The nature of the agency's goals and objectives
- The usefulness of a particular type of evaluation for the agency, its clientele, and the larger community
- The requirements of the funding source
- The extent of available resources (i.e., money, time, and staff)
- The political climate out of which the evaluation emerges

As can be surmised, home care evaluations, like evaluations of other human services, are shaped by a series of reality factors including both objective elements and subjective influences.

At its most fundamental level the home care evaluation entails an assessment of whether or not the agency's objectives have been accomplished in the time planned and with the resources allocated. It is best to perform such assessments at recurring points in time so that intended outcomes of services can be repeatedly compared against actual program outcomes. In this way the agency can determine at what points during the life of the organization, effectiveness, efficiency, impact, and so on, was greatest.

Home care assessments can seek answers to a variety of questions including:

1. *What was done?*

This approach is concerned with the amount of effort or input invested in the provision of service including number of personnel, amount of staff time, and both the quantity and quality of resources utilized.

2. *How was it done?*

This question addresses issues of process. The concern here is with coming up with an explanation for the ultimate results and is, therefore, an evaluation of the operations or inner workings of the home care agency.

3. *What took place?*

This approach focuses on the actual results of the invested effort. Evaluations of effect, performance, and impact are included here and are concerned with such variables as the number of home care clients served, changes in client condition or status, the extent to which institutionalization was avoided or delayed, and the degree to which clients were satisfied with the services provided.

4. *Did the results meet the need?*

Adequacy evaluations compare actual results against assessed need. In such an analysis the degree of achieved adequacy equals the degree to which program output satisfactorily met the level of need in the community. An evaluation of home care adequacy thus requires that an assessment of need for home care be performed as well as an evaluation of service results.

5. *At what cost were the results achieved?*

This is an evaluation of efficiency and focuses on an assessment of the implementation cost of delivering home care services in various ways. Funding sources are increasingly likely to expect home care programs to perform studies of this type.

Certain evaluation questions can be more easily and more rapidly answered than others. Traditionally, program evaluations in home care have tended to focus on measuring input, process, and output. Fewer studies of adequacy and efficiency have been carried out. Case practitioners will probably find the former to be more akin to their interests and experience.

Data collected for a home care evaluation can come from a variety of sources. Data sources potentially useful to the evaluator include: (a) agency service records and statistical reports, (b) informational surveys of clients served, (c) interviews with home care agency personnel, (d) interviews with experts in home care, (e) interviews with agency advisory boards, (f) participant and field observation data, (g) previously published home care research reports, and (h) records maintained by other home care programs.

It is usually a good idea to collect data from several sources when conducting evaluations. Varying the data collection methodology reduces dependence on any one source of data that may, alone, reflect bias in a particular direction. A good rule of thumb is to collect information that reflects the experience and points of view of both service providers (home care staff at all levels) and service recipients (home care clients and, when feasible, their significant others). Home care practitioners interested in reading further in the area of program evaluation are referred to texts by Patton (1982), Rossi and Freeman (1985), and Smith (1990).

4

Special Issues and Challenges

The successful practice of home health care requires continuous attention to a variety of issues and challenges relating to the process of program planning and service delivery. Effective provision of service is closely associated with the extent to which the activities of the home health service team reflect a philosophy of continuous collaboration, enlightened supervision, and general staff support. Effective program planning is increasingly tied to an appreciation for and expertise in marketing technique by those responsible for program development. These two special challenges—team cohesiveness and marketing expertise—in the field of home health care are the focus of this chapter.

The Home Health Team

Roles and Working Relationships

Home health care, by its very nature, creates an unusually heavy demand on the service team to work together in a collaborative manner. The challenge grows out of the intrinsic nature of the home health team combined with the unique structure and characteristics of home health care services. Unlike many interventive teams in the health and human services, home care teams are frequently composed of both professional and paraprofessional staff as well as an exceedingly wide range of disciplines that counts itself as a member of the group. In addition, the home health team rarely functions as a classical service unit delivering simultaneous services to the client or patient at approximately the same point in time. It is this variation in staff training and status as well as substantial differentiation in the timing of service provision by team members that make coordination and supervision so complex and challenging. The fact that home care clients frequently display an exceedingly wide range of physical and emotional problems speaks further to the importance of engaging a variety of social and health service professionals in the care plan.

Special concerns in addressing the issues of teams in home health care include:

1. Integrating and coordinating professional and paraprofessional staff (i.e., avoiding gaps and overlaps in services);
2. Bridging communication barriers due to use of discipline-specific jargon;
3. Bridging socioeconomic and cultural differences among staff;
4. Recognizing the need for leadership on the team and fulfilling the roles of "mediator" and "moderator" between staff;
5. Acknowledging and respecting professional turf and concomitant issues concerning authority;
6. Addressing issues of professional hierarchy (who trumps whom?) and interprofessional power struggles; and
7. Respecting the differences in skills and interests of team members.

Team practice in home health care carries with it the risk of conflict, competition, and poor coordination. The types of issues and concerns noted above must be resolved if the service package is to be properly delivered. All members need to make sure that in the final analysis the client's welfare takes precedence over interpersonal and interprofessional interests.

Good communication may indeed prove to be the pivotal key to successful team practice. Creative approaches to maintaining open lines of communication between members are critical. Team meetings and discussions should strive to reflect a generic or universal approach to information dissemination. That is, the "language" of the team should not be biased in its disciplinary orientation. Nurses, social workers, occupational and physical therapists, physicians, and aides should be made to feel equally at home with the terminology of team communication. Furthermore, team members should not rule out any and all conceivable methods for discussion and information dissemination. Both formal and informal approaches to having team members talk to each other are needed. These include: (a) case review conferences; (b) peer review meetings; (c) extensive use of telephone, memoranda, and in-person exchanges; (d) periodic team meetings; and (e) message sending to team members through team coordinators, leaders, and supervisors.

Supervision of Paraprofessionals

The case practitioner frequently will be assigned supervisory responsibility over home health aides, home attendants, homemakers, chore workers, and other paraprofessionals on the home health care team. Many of the principles that inform practice in professional supervision are applicable to paraprofessional supervision. Home care supervision has been defined as

> the means by which an agency assures itself, the community and the policy body that its programs and services are provided in the most effective and efficient manner. As a process, supervision is the means by which workers are helped to perform the jobs for which they will be held accountable. (National HomeCaring Council, 1982)

Home care supervisors function to encourage staff accountability, increase coordination, and promote effective implementation of the service plan. To perform these functions effectively the supervisor should have: (a) considerable knowledge and expertise in direct service delivery to the frail and homebound elderly; (b) a thorough understanding of the home health care agency's policies and procedures; and (c) advanced skills in communication, training, organizational process, and problem solving.

Paraprofessional supervision encompasses at least three potential dimensions of central responsibility:

1. Management and administration,
2. Education and training, and
3. Support.

Kadushin (1985) has endorsed a similar categorization of functional responsibilities for the social work supervisor. The administrative or managerial home care supervisor may be involved in any and all of the following tasks:

1. Staff recruitment and selection;
2. Inducting and placing the worker;
3. Work planning;
4. Work assignments;
5. Work delegation;
6. Monitoring, reviewing, evaluating work;
7. Coordinating work;
8. The communication function;
9. The supervisor as administrative buffer; and
10. The supervisor as change agent (Kadushin, 1985).

It should be clear from the above that in-depth knowledge of the inner workings of the home care agency including its structure, characteristics, and problems, will be essential if the case practitioner is to discharge successfully the responsibilities of administrative supervisor. The capacity to monitor and evaluate the work performance of the home health aide or homemaker also requires a thorough understanding of the circumstances pertaining to a particular case assignment. Of course each agency will determine the range of administrative tasks to be assumed by any single supervisor. At the least, supervisors will probably assume the responsibility for scheduling and tracking the amount of staff effort expended on each case.

The educational or training supervisor is primarily oriented to building up the scope and breadth of skills and expertise of the paraprofessional. By offering comments on materials and ideas presented by the paraprofessional during the supervisory session, the supervisor focuses in on teaching supervisees to deal successfully with the following particularly demanding elements of home health care service delivery:

- Establishing trusting client relationships
- Being attuned to evidence of sudden change in client status
- Successfully accessing community resources
- Maintaining appropriate worker-client-significant other relations
- Understanding the dynamics of the client's informal support system
- Coping with the personal stress associated with home health care service provision

Educational supervision is a function that must not be overlooked in working with paraprofessionals. In fact the opportunity it provides for them to grow and mature in their work may be one of the greatest rewards of engagement in this field of service for supervisor and supervisee alike. In the process workers are taught how to do their jobs effectively.

Successful educational supervision in home health care requires that the supervisee be motivated to learn and that he or she be able to direct a good amount of energy to the task. Furthermore, learning expectations on the part of the supervisor and supervisee should be pitched to a level that is mutually agreed upon and attainable. In a sense, then, educational expectations need to be individually tailored to the interests and capacities of the participating paraprofessional. The educational process should also be an interactive one—one in which the worker participates in his or her own learning and is not simply lectured to. It should also have practical application—that is, the supervisee should have the opportunity to test out what he or she has learned in the workplace. Of course the supervisor has the responsibility to present educational and training content in a positive, meaningful, organized, and understandable fashion.

Workers in the field of home care can expect their full share of job-related stress and strain. Employee stress is closely related to the emotional demands associated with working with vulnerable, functionally impaired adults in the intimate confines of their homes. Case practitioner supervisors should therefore always be attuned to these stress factors and should accordingly provide the necessary support to their paraprofessional staff. Supportive supervision is, however, different from personal therapy, the latter function being one that is inappropriate and places the supervisor in a potentially precarious position.

Supportive supervision is concerned with expressive considerations (Kadushin, 1985). Supervision in home care that focuses on support should be particularly concerned with identifying the source of job-related stress or tension (e.g., the client, another worker, the assignment, the agency and its policies, supervision itself, etc.) and then implementing strategies that allow for the alleviation of those feelings. Supportive supervision may therefore seek to bring change in the worker or in the surrounding environment. In other words, supervisory support can entail a process that enables the worker to learn to accept a situation or condition that is unalterable (e.g., restrictive agency eligibility criteria or service coverage) or it may entail efforts to bring about an actual change in the circumstances that served to bring about the stressful feelings in the first place (e.g., taking a worker off a particularly difficult case or intervening on behalf of a worker to resolve a disagreement with another staff person).

Supportive supervisory techniques tend to focus on helping clients deal with negative feelings of one sort or another. Being available, an empathic orientation, patient listening, creating opportunities for ventilation, reassurance or confirmation of a worker's decisions, and recognizing those frustrations that are universally felt by others can all serve to reduce stress and discontent among staff. Active intervention on the part of the supervisor in order to alter an undesirable condition should be considered when appropriate as well as arranging for opportunities for team and peer group ventilation and problem-solving meetings.

Of course home health care supervisors may assume a variety of roles during the course of their work. These include advocate, change agent, consultant, monitor, helper, self-assessor, and enforcer. For a review of these functions see Austin (1981).

Figure 4.1 outlines a series of classic dos and don'ts for the home health care practice supervisor.

In-Service Training and Continuing Education

An ongoing program of in-service training for staff at all levels of the home care organization as well as periodic opportunities to attend in-house and community continuing education programs and conferences is essential. Educational opportunities represent one of the few payoffs assured to workers who have committed themselves to this field of service. Skills enhancement reduces the likelihood of staff burnout, acknowledges the valuable role that the staff play in home health care, and prepares staff for advancement in the organization and in their careers.

Appropriate basic training also guards against the dangers of doing harm both to your clients and yourself during the course of service provision (Moore & Layzer, 1983). Skill is required in providing "hands-on" care to the homebound, preparing special diets, transferring clients from one location to another, performing accurate assessments and reassessments, and counseling in crisis situa-

DO:

Be aware of different learning styles among supervisees

Use varied approaches to supervision (e.g., direct presentation of information, examples, role playing, reading, audiovisual aides, discussion, brainstorming)

Be aware of supervisee's existing knowledge and skills and gaps in same

Communicate in a fashion that is understood (e.g., proper level of diction, etc.)

Encourage queries and feedback

Be aware of supervisee's perspective from his or her vantage point in the hierarchy

Be aware of supervisee's personality and sensitivities and tailor supervision accordingly

Take responsibility for supervisee's performance by supporting and helping him or her advance

DON'T:

Be autocratic—learning, teaching, and evaluation are mutual processes

Be condescending

Automatically reject opinions that differ from your own. Be willing to discuss; this does not diminish your status, rather, it increases respect

Pass judgment on their person, but rather on their behavior (e.g., Don't say "You're a lazy person," say "In your work with our agency, you only have done the minimum amount of work necessary")

Reject criticism of yourself by staff. Supervisees are entitled to their opinions.

Allow personal feelings—good or bad—about staff to influence your professional relationship with them

---

Figure 4.1. The DOs and DON'Ts of Home Health Care Practice Supervision

tions. Furthermore, training is a basic requirement under the federal Medicare Conditions of Participation for Medicare and Medicaid reimbursed home care agencies.

As noted by Austin (1981), training content in organizational settings can be categorized into three main areas: (a) functional skills, (b) specific content skills, and (c) adaptive skills. Functional skills refer to the capacity of staff to perform particular agency tasks and functions. Content skills refer to competencies required to deliver agency services in the required manner. Adaptive skills involve those competencies that staff are required to display in managing their own behavior in response to agency change and conformity as well as the nature of the agency's physical work environment.

Of course, to varying degrees, persons entering the field of home health care bring with them some of the functional, content, and adaptive competencies required of practice. These are obtained through various experiences, including early childhood relations with parents and other role models; peer relations; elementary, secondary, and college education; and graduate- and professional-level

Skills Area	Subject
Functional	How to perform the home health intake
	Conducting the home care assessment
	Techniques of home care counseling
	Diagnosing change in the homebound client
	Legal issues in home care
	Safety in the home
	Working with the sensory-impaired client
	Death, dying, and bereavement
	Updates on change in federal, state, and local home care policy
	Legislative developments and home care advocacy technique
	New technology in home health care services
	The alcoholic client
	Working with the Alzheimer's patient
Content	Orientation to personnel practices
	Using agency forms correctly
	Reviewing agency policy and procedure
	Maintaining accurate agency records
	Working with computerized information support systems in home health care
	Techniques for referral file maintenance
	Home care service planning and development
Adaptive	Techniques for stress management
	Effective time management
	Communication skills in the workplace
	Decision making during a crisis
	Promoting coordination and teamwork on the job
	Managing staff relationships
	Interdisciplinary networking in the agency
	Dynamics of advisory board and committee operations

Figure 4.2. Training Subjects for Home Health Care Agency Staff

training. Some training content, however, will not have been secured prior to employment. In-service, on-the-job training combined with opportunities for staff to attend community continuing education programs and educational conferences serve to fill the gap. The need for such opportunities is just as important for paraprofessional as professional staff. The differences lie purely in the focus and intensity of the training content. Figure 4.2 reflects the range of training material that might be considered for staff in home health care agencies in refining functional, content, and adaptive skills.

The many skills and the knowledge base associated with the provision of home health care services are outlined in the appendix and organized as model fieldwork assignments. While the primary intent of the fieldwork assignments is to help students maximize their learning in fieldwork opportunities in the home health care setting, the assignments can also be used in helping to educate and supervise new home health personnel.

Case practitioners in home care should be prepared to assume the role of trainer in the agency. Few organizations can afford to hire individuals who assume sole responsibility for in-service education. As a result, case practitioners are frequently turned to because of their professional training and supervisory expertise. According to Kirschner and Rosengarten (1982), the role of educator naturally combines with a series of other functional roles including negotiator, advocate, diagnostician, therapist, and home manager. The professional case practitioner becomes a natural source of training expertise due to his or her knowledge of such issues as the psychology of somatic illness, psychogeriatrics, personality theories, ego psychology, family dynamics, crisis intervention, community resources, and government entitlements (Kirschner & Rosengarten, 1982).

Several important points should be kept in mind when organizing agency in-services:

1. *Target your population.* Make a determination whether in-services will be geared to interdisciplinary versus discipline-specific audiences, professional versus paraprofessional staff. Certain in-services may be better focused on a very delineated, specific audience, while others will have relevance to agency staff as a whole. The nature of the topic combined with demands on time will influence your decision.

2. *Keep abreast of new developments.* Training personnel in the home care agency should always be on the lookout for service innovations, policy changes, and research discoveries about which staff should know. Similarly, trainers should have some mechanism whereby they are kept apprised of internal agency issues and needs as well as special staff concerns that can be addressed by means of an in-service. A training advisory committee comprised of staff, administrative personnel, and consumer representatives can be extremely helpful in planning in-service and continuing education programs for the agency.

3. *Don't overwhelm your staff.* Effective training programs require careful planning. In-services should be properly sequenced such that new staff have an opportunity to orient themselves to the agency before being exposed to detailed educational materials. Relevancy of training is critical as well. Material presented should be meaningful to staff, having direct application to their work responsibilities and functions.

4. *Remember that people learn differently.* Agency training programs should be sensitive to the wide range of approaches to learning. Among the methods trainers can utilize successfully in the field of home health are lectures, audiovisual materials, role playing, discussions, simulations, and videotaping. Distributing handouts at each session is especially important in order that staff can, at their leisure, quickly refer back to specific concepts and ideas that were discussed. Dynamic presentations that emphasize learning by doing are likely to have the greatest impact.

5. *Encourage staff participation.* Home care workers should be encouraged not only to attend on-the-job training programs but also to take responsibility for gathering and/or presenting materials at the sessions themselves. Workers can assist in such tasks as collecting resource materials, identifying and inviting community speakers, preparing handouts, researching specialized topics, keeping abreast of training programs offered elsewhere in the community, and even assuming the role of trainer at specified times. Encouraging mutual responsibility for learning in the agency will better ensure the establishment of a loyal and motivated audience.

Home health agencies would be wise to maintain an up-to-date library of catalogues and bulletins describing recent educational and training films and videotapes addressing issues of aging, care in the home, and personnel development. Utilizing audiovisual materials and subsequent discussion for in-service training can represent a refreshing and effective departure from the customary approaches of training staff. Many film distributors and production companies now specialize in topical areas related to home care. Consider also the utilization of audiovisual equipment as part of the training sequence itself. Allowing staff at all levels to role play difficult worker-client situations on film creates an excellent vehicle for the critical review of staff practice.

Film Distributors That Specialize in Aging- and Health-Related Films

AARP A/V Programs
Program Scheduling Office
Program Resources Department
601 E Street, NW
Washington, DC 20049

Carle Medical Communications
510 West Main Street
Urbana, IL 61801
Tel: (217) 384-4838

Filmakers Library
124 East 40th Street
New York, NY 10016
Tel: (212) 808-4980
Fax: (212) 808-4983

Films for the Humanities & Sciences
P.O. Box 2053
Princeton, NJ 08543-2053
Tel: (800) 257-5126; (609) 452-1128
Fax: (609) 452-1602

Insight Media
121 West 85th Street
New York, NY 10024
Tel: (212) 721-6316
Fax: (212) 799-5309

Milner-Fenwick, Inc.
2125 Greenspring Drive
Timonium, MD 21093
Tel: (301) 252-1700; (800) 638-8652

Phoenix Films, Inc.
468 Park Avenue South, 10th Floor
New York, NY 10016
Tel: (212) 684-5910; (800) 221-1274

International Tele-Film Enterprises
47 Densley Avenue
Toronto, Ontario M6M5A8
Tel: (416) 241-4483

Pyramid Film and Video
Box 1048
Santa Monica, CA 90406-1048
Tel: (800) 421-2304
(310) 828-7577 (in California)

Spectrum Films, Inc.
2755 Jefferson Street, Suite 103
Carlsbad, CA 92008-9965
Tel: (619) 434-6191

Terra Nova Films
9848 S. Winchester Avenue
Chicago, IL 60643
Tel: (312) 881-8491

University Film & Video
University of Minnesota
1313 Fifth Street, S.E., Suite 108
Minneapolis, MN 55414
Tel: (800) 542-0013 (in-state)
(800) 847-8251 (out-of-state)

Video Services
Department of Physical Therapy
University of Maryland
School of Medicine
32 South Greene Street
Baltimore, MD 21201
Tel: (301) 328-5497; (301) 328-7720

The Continuing Education Program*
School of Social Welfare
State University of New York at Albany
135 Western Avenue
Albany, NY 12222

*Produces and distributes videotape and film training resources on such issues as communication, how-to-run meetings, job management skills, supervision/leadership, evaluation and training. Also available are videotape-film packages addressing the special interview skills required of Medicaid application workers, client assessment, interviewing, client goal planning, home safety and management, food and nutrition, working with families, the blind client and more.

The following organizations may be able to provide home care agencies with additional useful materials for in-service training seminars and continuing education workshops. The National Home-Caring Council has, in particular, developed a model curriculum for homemakers and home health aides based on approximately 75 hours of classroom and laboratory instruction as well as field practice. The council also has developed practical training materials that can be utilized by staff engaged in home health care service supervision, administration, and management.

The National Association for Home Health Care (NAHC), a not-for-profit trade association representing home care agencies and hospices, sponsors educational and professional development programs and has developed a wide range of training publications. NAHC also publishes a comprehensive resource directory of the nation's home care and hospice providers.

National Organizations That Accredit Home Care Services

National HomeCaring Council
235 Park Avenue South
New York, NY 10003
(212) 674-4990

National League for Nursing
American Public Health Association
10 Columbus Circle
New York, NY 10019
(212) 582-1022

Joint Commission on Accreditation of Health Care Organizations
875 North Michigan Avenue
Chicago, IL 60611
(312) 642-6061

Other National Home Care Organizations

American Hospital Association
Division of Ambulatory and Home Care Services
840 North Lake Shore Drive
Chicago, IL 60611
(312) 280-6000

Home Health Services and Staffing Association
2101 L Street, N.W.
Washington, DC 20037
(202) 775-4707

National Association for Home Care
519 C Street, N.E.
Washington, DC 20002-5809
(202) 547-7424

National Organizations With Related Interests

American Association of Retired Persons
601 E Street, N.W.
Washington, DC 20049

American Association of Homes and Services for the Aging
1129 20th Street, N.W., Suite 400
Washington, DC 20036
(202) 296-5960

The Gerontological Society of America
1275 K Street, N.W., Suite 350
Washington, DC 20005-4006
(202) 842-1275

National Association of Social Workers
750 First Street, N.E.
Washington, DC, 20002-4241
(202) 408-8600

National Council on Aging, Inc.
600 Maryland Avenue, S.W., West Wing 100
Washington, DC 20024
(202) 479-1200

American Society on Aging
833 Market Street, Suite 516
San Francisco, CA 94103
(415) 543-2617

Center for Understanding Aging
Framingham State College
Framingham, MA 01701
(508) 626-4979

Marketing Expertise and Strategies: Marketing Home Care

What does marketing have to do with delivering home health care services? At first glance very little. Consider, however, the following undeniable trends:

1. America is aging. Approximately 13% of the population is 65 years of age or older. The fastest-growing segment of the United States population comprises those adults 75 years and older—the elderly cohort most likely to be experiencing physical and functional decline and, consequently, a need for community services.

2. The aged are a powerful force in the marketplace today. Their economic status has been improving at a particularly rapid pace during the past 20 years, and they currently have more discretionary spending power than any other segment of the American population.

3. The expectations of the elderly population are changing. A more sophisticated and informed aged cohort brings with them heightened expectations concerning the availability of a variety of service options. Increased service options bring with them the reality of competition and many of the characteristics of the traditional business world. In order to stay ahead of the game, new services need to be developed.

4. Home care agencies, like any other organizations, need to be concerned with organizational survival and the sustained well-being of their staff. The absence of assurances that public resources will, in all cases, successfully meet the costs of home care services creates increasing demands on agencies to search out alternative sources of financial security. Such a perspective is essential if you are to have any degree of control over your fate as an organizational entity. Results of a national study of executive directors of health and social service organizations (including home health care agencies) indicate that marketing initiatives are now commonplace activities and result in increased financial security for the organization and greater assurance of adequate enrollment (Kaye & Reisman, 1991a).

Home care marketing as a philosophy and set of methodological skills confronts the above trends head on. It aims to optimize agency growth and success by defining the role your organization can play in light of the expressed needs and demands of the elder marketplace. A marketing perspective requires home care agency staff to think creatively. Clients are viewed as consumers and other home care agencies as competitors. Maintaining consumer enrollment in your agency is tantamount to agency survival.

What Is Marketing?

It is easier to determine what marketing is not than to define what marketing is. Marketing is different from selling. The primary focus of marketing is on consumer needs (i.e., selling that for which people express a need), whereas selling focuses exclusively on the available service or product (i.e.., sell what you have regardless of consumer need). Marketing is a process that utilizes an array of techniques including research, planning, R&D (research and development), advertising, distribution, and so on. On the other hand, selling relies primarily upon advertising, public relations, and networking.

Marketing and selling make use of quite different financial strategies as well. While marketing aims to increase revenues or service enrollment through consumer satisfaction, the goal of selling is to increase revenues through volume. In essence, marketing is more consumer-centered than product-centered. In addition, marketing differs from public relations in that marketing is quantifiable. Public relations is merely one component or stage in the marketing process. In general, marketing implies a willingness to meet the consumers halfway after working toward a better understanding of who they are and how their needs can be met. And marketing should be an ongoing process, not a one-time effort carried out at the point of program initiation because the consumer market is always changing.

Marketing includes a number of discrete components including the following:

1. *Market Research.* During this phase in the marketing process, information is collected about both the internal and external environment of the proposed home health care organization. External issues of concern include identifying need, gauging existing home care services/competition, tracking health and functional impairment trends, assessing available funding/resources, assessing the level of risk, and describing your target population. Internal issues of concern include assessments of the capacity and adequacy of the physical plant, staff, equipment, capital, referral network, board, and government relations. This step in the process may be preceded by a feasibility study (needs assessment) in order to determine whether the project is likely to be viable at the outset. This preliminary step can save the home care planner much time and money.

2. *Market Planning.* This stage provides the framework for identifying, collecting, and capturing select segments of the home care marketplace. For example, it is at this point that a determination may be made to expand the program to include hospice care or adult day care because market research indicated significant need in these areas.

3. *Marketing Strategy Development.* This phase entails a commitment to new service development based upon results of the first two phases. It also includes taking advantage of existing opportunities and gaps in the marketplace. Thus it is at this point that additional services are developed that were not initially contemplated (e.g., developing an adult day care program, a hospice project, or transportation services).

4. *Advertising.* This activity differs from public relations in that it refers to the use of *paid* communications to influence the home care market. Decisions are made concerning the relative use of broadcast versus print media at this time.

5. *Public Relations.* This refers primarily to *free* publicity to promote goodwill within the community toward your service. Staff involvement on community boards, advisory committees of other agencies, interagency councils, and so on, can go far to further a positive view of the agency's mission. Becoming involved in community issues that may not be immediately related to home care service delivery is also strategic at this point in order that a wide range of potentially fruitful contacts and supporters be nurtured.

6. *Fund Development.* This phase includes the active solicitation of funding for the organization. Home care marketing strategy at this stage can include investigations into the availability of both public and private funds.

7. *Consumer Relations or Liaison.* It is critical to identify an individual who will act as an intermediary between the service provider (the home care program) and the consumers or potential consumers (the elderly clients and their significant others). This will serve to better ensure ongoing positive relations and image within the community.

8. *Sales.* This refers to the point in the process where you "close" or complete the marketing process through enrollment of clients in the program.

As one moves through the various stages of marketing the service, a series of pivotal questions should be answered. They include:

What business is the home care program in?
Who are the program's clients and what kinds of needs do they have?
What are the major strengths and weaknesses of your home care program?
Who are the major competitors with whom you must reckon?
Which potential client groups in the community offer the best opportunities for the home care agency?
What strategies should be developed to maintain an effective community service?
How can you keep abreast of changes in need within the home care service population?

Marketing and the Case Practitioner

The case practitioner plays an important role in the marketing process. Consider the following:

1. The practitioner has direct access to clients and is the employee most likely to receive consumer feedback. Be aware of the value of this information in the ongoing marketing process and share the information with administrators. Client feedback may provide data critical in clarifying who your target population is and also who your competitors are as well as the major gaps in the home care marketplace.

2. Out in the community the case practitioner is, in effect, performing a public relations function. The practitioner has continuous contact with staff in other community programs as they carry out the information and referral function. The view that community agencies develop of any particular home care agency is primarily influenced by the experience they have had interacting with front line providers.

3. The case practitioner often has primary responsibility for consumer relations and serves as consumer liaison between service provider and market. On occasion the case practitioner may assume the role of ombudsperson or mediator, resolving disagreements between client and agency as he or she is called on to interpret agency policy and procedure in the context of client need.

4. Because of the practitioner's direct role in home care, that person may be in the best position to think creatively about service modification and development. Administrators, in reality, are often far removed from information concerning the service experience and client need, and it is sensitivity to this type of information that is needed for effective marketing. This is why administrators so often hire consultants to conduct the marketing analysis. Case practitioners can be an important source for consultation even if they do not possess the expertise required for actual programs planning and development.

5. The case practitioner is well aware of the characteristics of the client's informal network and therefore can be counted among those best able to recognize appropriate targets for marketing (the elderly themselves may not be your primary target, but, rather, their informal and formal supports).

In actuality, the marketing process in home health care is not unrelated to the process of program planning and development. Indeed both utilize related methodology. The primary difference may well lie in variations of philosophy and emphasis. (For further discussion of the marketing process as it pertains to the home care intake and screening process see Chapter 5. Chapter 3 deals with the methodology of program development and design.)

5

Intake/Screening

This chapter considers the initial phases of geriatric case practice in home health care. It focuses on the requirements for conducting effective community outreach, client screening, and intake. Consideration of specialized screening technique in home health care is also addressed, including procedures for determining client eligibility, appropriateness of care, information gathering, maintaining confidentiality, and conducting initial home visits. Finally, the basic components of a home care client intake form are identified.

Conducting Effective Community Outreach

Home health care agencies do not have the luxury of accepting for service all applicants in need of assistance in their homes. Agency eligibility criteria frequently differ from one program to the next. These criteria for service eligibility are in large part determined by such factors as the nature of the target population, agency auspice and mission, agency location, and funding or reimbursement source requirements. The strategies and methods employed in conducting home health care community outreach should be, in large part, shaped by this set of agency eligibility policies:

1. *Targeting Your Population.* The characteristics of the service population to be served by a particular agency is heavily influenced

by that organization's mandate or mission. A community hospital that decides to implement a home health care program is probably going to abide by past tradition and expertise in terms of the range and types of services offered and clients served. If that hospital had established a name for itself as a provider of intensive, acute care services including nursing, physical therapy, speech therapy, and health counseling assistance, it can be expected to continue to concentrate on offering such services in the older person's home. Similarly, home health aide services are more likely to supplement these services than those of the friendly visitor, chore worker, or home attendant. On the other hand, a family service agency in the community will more likely focus on providing a range of social support services for its home care clients such as personal and family counseling, homemaker, housekeeping, and shopping services, and telephone reassurance.

In each case above, the population you ultimately target for agency outreach should be the one that will most likely need and benefit from the range of personnel and services you are able to offer, whether these reflect a medical or health emphasis, a social support emphasis, or some combination of the two. Specific eligibility criteria that should be considered in conducting outreach that is sensitive to an agency's mission include: (a) the older person's age, (b) the older person's financial status (including his or her eligibility for or coverage by third-party payments), (c) the older person's geographic location (he or she needs to fall within the neighborhood boundaries serviced by the agency program), (d) the availability or absence of family members and other potential informal supports such as friends and neighbors (some programs serve only those elderly who are without immediately available relatives), and (e) the nature and degree of disability or illness evidenced by the older person (programs may establish a cutoff point in terms of disability below or above which they are unable to accept an applicant for service).

2. *Recruitment and Outreach.* It is usually a good rule of thumb not to depend on any single method of recruitment when conducting agency outreach. Rather, it is best to utilize a variety of formal and informal approaches reflecting both personalized and more broad or mass appeals in the community. It is also critical to keep in mind that a great many of the older people who are likely to be in need of home health care services are apt to be rather isolated. Partially and

completely homebound older adults are frequently counted among the "invisible elderly," that is, they are not known to the formal service agency network. Therefore, agency outreach would do well to emphasize both formal and informal avenues of communication when publicizing their presence and service offerings.

Formal avenues of communication include notifications distributed to community social service agencies, physicians, hospitals, and government offices (e.g., General Social Services, Social Security, legal services for the frail elderly, community mental health centers, senior centers, etc.). Informal routes include contact with local community clergy, neighbors, friends, relatives, neighborhood merchants, landlords, self-help organizations, family support and respite groups, and so on.

Outreach strategies that have been effectively utilized by home health agencies include: ads in local newspapers; notices on community bulletin boards in libraries, churches and synagogues, senior centers, community luncheon clubs, and grocery stores; and announcements sent to community organizations serving the elderly and disabled such as family service agencies, casework services, hospitals and medical centers, nursing homes and homes for the aged. Individualized visits and presentations at senior citizen centers and community clubs for older adults as well as social service agencies and local doctors offices may be worthwhile as well even though they can be time consuming. Contact with the growing network of professionals in private geriatric case practice and management may also be worthwhile as these professionals are frequently a rich source of ongoing referrals.

3. *The Nature of Agency Auspice.* The degree of need to engage in extensive agency outreach and recruitment will depend greatly upon agency auspice. For example, a proprietary (for-profit) agency must do more outreach than a Medicaid vendor, public program, or voluntary organization because its fees are higher and there is no natural referral system from which it is able to benefit. In addition, there is currently considerable competition among private home care agencies due to a glut in the market in many communities.

4. *Agency Location.* Agency location is an additional factor determining the extent to which outreach is required as well as the methods best employed in carrying out recruitment. In rural communities

where home care services are frequently few and far between, minimal recruitment is needed. One must only make the agency's purpose and presence known. There is no need to compete. On the other hand, in large cosmopolitan areas the opposite is generally the rule. Urban, inner-city areas and suburban settings may be largely saturated with a wide variety of home health care services. In such settings, unless you are a subsidized service entity, you will likely need to engage competitively for clients. Strategies in such settings may include paid advertisements in newspapers, special arrangements with private practitioners whereby clients are referred to the agency for a "finders fee," and sophisticated marketing approaches, including seductive literature and extensive use of the electronic media.

Marketing, Competition, and Home Health Care

The home care market is a burgeoning one. No longer serving only the Medicare patient in need of acute, short-term skilled nursing care, competition within the home care network encompasses the delivery of traditional medical home health services, support services, high-tech services, home care equipment, case management, and so on (Boothe, 1986). Increases in competition have led in turn to the employment of increasingly sophisticated techniques for marketing home care services. Within the same community large-scale home care companies serving hundreds of clients a day are operating alongside small-scale programs with caseloads of only several dozen individuals. The ability to function in such a highly competitive setting is becoming an essential skill in order to ensure agency survival.

Joanne Meany-Handy (1986) perceives this change in the home care market to be reflective of a movement toward practices that are common to traditional business markets. While highly technical marketing strategies will not be needed nor appropriate for many home care programs, this type of approach should be seriously considered in highly competitive communities. If marketing is perceived as encompassing all those activities that an agency engages in to educate and recruit its target population and develop needed services, the objectives of marketing in home health care naturally follow:

- generating revenues through the development and utilization of income-producing services
- assuring that services reach people who need them
- meeting the intense competition in the field
- building an image for the organization
- achieving continued growth of the services and organization (Meany-Handy, 1986).

If a marketing approach appears appropriate for a particular home care program, then one should consider the following activities: (a) conducting market research, (b) selecting target markets, (c) identifying the service mix, (d) selecting strategies for each market segment, and (e) developing and implementing the marketing plan.

A variety of books that present highly detailed approaches to health care marketing are available. They include: *Marketing Management, Analysis Planning and Control* (Kotler, 1980), *Health Care Marketing* (Cooper, 1979), and *Marketing Health Care* (MacStravic, 1977).

Initial Screening and Intake

Client intake or screening is usually viewed as the initial service-management function of geriatric case practice in home health care. Intake procedures may be carried out during an initial in-home assessment, an office visit by the client and/or his or her relatives, by means of telephone interview, or some combination of the above. The National HomeCaring Council, Inc. (1982) defines intake as a twofold process:

1. It is the process through which individuals seek services. A potential recipient may have someone help gain access to a service agency or needed component.

2. Intake is also the process through which the service agency seeks to identify the individuals and families in the community that it can serve.

Agency intake can also be visualized as the first phase in a sequence of stages along the client pathway to home care services (Kaye, 1985a). The home care client pathway encompasses the following discrete stages:

1. Intake/Screening
2. Needs Assessment
3. Case Planning
4. Service Delivery
5. Monitoring/Evaluation

(Stages 2 through 5 are discussed in subsequent chapters.)

The older person can reach intake, the entry point to service, in a variety of ways. Awareness of a particular home care service may have been arrived at through self-referral or by means of the assistance of a relative, friend, neighbor, family physician, hospital, or social service agency. Earlier outreach and recruitment efforts may also result in the discovery of an older person who is homebound and has not yet made an effective linkage with the service network.

In general the stage of intake entails an initial determination concerning the appropriateness of the referral and whether the older person is likely to satisfy the home care program's eligibility criteria. Ineligible applicants are referred elsewhere, whereas eligible persons are able to move to the next stage along the client pathway—that of needs assessment.

Determination of Eligibility

Regardless of the source of referral (self-referral or referral from the formal or informal support network of that older person) eligibility must be carefully assessed. The intake or screening worker should never assume that the referring party has, prior to referral, made such an assessment appropriately. It is important to remember that referring parties may have a powerful stake in successfully completing what is, in fact, an inappropriate referral for service (i.e., it could enable them to "dump" a problematic or difficult client or increase their own referral statistics to satisfy their funding source).

Determination of eligibility is generally based upon a rather specific set of criteria established by the home care agency, its funding source, and/or government mandate. These eligibility criteria are made concrete by means of an agency intake form. Fact-finding activities by the intake worker should include the gathering of information from as many available sources as possible. If the older person is mentally capable of providing all or even a minute portion of the requisite information, it is imperative that the worker tap this source first. Failing to do so is, in effect, sending the older adult one or more insulting messages—"because you are old, your knowledge of yourself and your needs is unimportant;" "I am negating your existence by not addressing you directly;" "I am conspiring behind your back with your friends, relatives, and other service providers to make decisions concerning *your* life and you may have no say in the matter."

After gathering information from the potential client, as much supplemental information as possible should be gathered from other service providers who currently (or previously) provide assistance to the potential client and, when available, from family, friends, and significant others.

One may, at times, be placed in the position of detective when the information from two or more sources is in conflict. There are several steps that can be taken in such a situation. First, determine whether the information in question is purely factual (e.g., a social security number, date of birth, or amount of social security benefits) or a matter of a point of view or opinion (e.g., emotional stability of the client, mental clarity, degree of infirmity). In the event of disagreement in terms of factual data, one simply must go to an authoritative source for documentation (e.g., obtaining the award letter from the Social Security Administration indicating both the applicant's social security number and amount of check; a marriage certificate or citizenship papers indicating date of birth).

When the conflictual information is of a subjective nature, one has a more challenging task, often accompanied by an ethical dilemma. First, double check all sources of information that are at odds in order that those parties may check their information again and perhaps alter their point of view. Simply learning who or what is the source of their information may help you in determining its reliability. If the "double check" method does not prove fruitful, and all sources stand by their information, the worker is placed in the position of passing judgment on the issue. One must carefully weigh the reliability of the sources, consider their potential stake, if any, in providing misinformation, and make a personal evaluation based upon the balance of information provided and any first-hand knowledge of the potential client. In all circumstances, even when all sources concur, it is important to evaluate information critically and not to accept it on face value. Above all, remember that there is a professional responsibility to the older person. The bottom line is quality care to the client when the worker, supported by adequate documentation, believes it is appropriate. You are a service provider with the client's best interest in mind, not a court of law.

Determination of Appropriateness

A second consideration in the intake process is that of appropriateness. This factor differs from eligibility because it is based upon judgment concerning client welfare rather than on meeting eligibility requirements. An individual may indeed satisfy eligibility criteria, but alternate care may be preferable. The worker has an ethical responsibility to inform the potential client of all such alternatives that are appropriate and available. For example, Miss Fletcher meets the requirements for home care services: she has some minor physical and sensory impairments (arthritis, glaucoma, and requires a hearing aid), is financially limited, and desires home care because she cannot go out of her home, which is in a crime-ridden neighborhood. She has been repeatedly victimized and has already suffered a broken arm and has many cuts and bruises from the most recent assault. Although Miss Fletcher does satisfy all eligibility criteria for your home care agency, you know that she would also be eligible for the Section 202 housing project located in a safer section of town. In such a situation you have a professional responsibility to inform the older person of this alternative, especially since this option may be more likely to satisfy her needs. It then, of course, is left to Miss Fletcher to decide which type of care suits her best.

Information Gathering Techniques

The manner in which data are collected from a potential client is of paramount importance. One must have sensitivity to the individual's emotional state during application for care as well as to his or her possible mental and sensory impairments that may hinder the data collection process.

While for the worker an intake may just be one event during a busy day, for the applicant it holds much greater significance. It may represent a significant concession to the increasing number of infirmities of old age; an unwelcome reminder that total independence is no longer feasible; and the discomfort, in some cases, of having to depend on what is perceived to be "charity" or a "handout" (a concept that is totally abhorrent to the current generation of elders).

In addition, the intake interview may take place in the home care agency, in a hospital, or somewhere else that is unfamiliar turf to the older person. Sensitivity to these feelings and their related needs is crucial.

While only a small proportion of the elderly have marked mental, physical, or sensory deficits, many of those seeking home care services have done so because of such impairments. These can make information collection a slow and frustrating process for both the worker and the potential client. If the worker airs his or her frustration and annoyance, the client can be expected to grow even more upset, thereby slowing the process even further. To assist in promoting a timely and sensitive intake process:

1. *Be Patient.* Allow the client to set a pace that is in accordance with his or her own ability. The client may well be unable to respond at the same pace at which you are able to pose the questions.

2. *Listen Carefully,* even if what is being related to you does not seem to be relevant to the topic at hand. If you stop the person, he or she may not "hear" subsequent questions, wanting to convey that which he or she had been unable to communicate earlier.

3. *Speak Up.* If the person is hearing impaired, it is essential that you speak loudly and clearly, looking directly at the individual so that he or she is able to see your lips.

4. *Read Out Loud.* If the person is visually impaired, remember that you may need to read all written material out loud, twice if necessary for full comprehension.

5. *Listen Patiently.* In the event that the applicant has a speech impairment or is aphasic, listen patiently and be understanding. Do not try to complete the applicant's sentence before he or she does. Wait for the person to finish the sentence, and then, if there is doubt as to what was said, repeat the sentence as a question. (e.g., Miss Russo states unclearly, "I was born in 1909 in Ohio." Worker: "Oh, so you were born right here in Ohio in 1909?" Miss Russo: "Yes.") This allows the worker to gather accurate personal data and prevents the client with a speech impediment from feeling inadequate or self-conscious regarding his or her disability.

6. *Address the Client Directly.* The mentally impaired individual will most likely be accompanied by a significant other who will assist in the provision of information. Keep in mind that the mentally impaired person experiences normal emotions and should be treated with the dignity and respect afforded others. Regardless of the degree of impairment, always address questions to the older adult applying for service. Allow an opportunity for the applicant to reply. If he or she is unable to do so adequately, you may then address the client's companion. In all cases keep in mind that you are often requesting information of a personal nature and that sensitivity to this fact is important.

It is helpful to question in a conversational context rather than "cross-examining" by shooting one question after the next. In addition, it can be helpful to allow the person to answer questions in an order other than that which appears on the intake form. If the older person begins to share information that appears in a later section of the form because it is easier for him or her to share such material, allow the person to do so. You can always return to missing data at a later point in the interview. Ann Burack-Weiss and Frances Coyle Brennan (1984) have prepared an extremely useful manual for the practitioner responsible for performing or supervising agency intakes or "first encounters" as they describe the process. The background and context of "first encounters" are established as is the process of obtaining and using information and setting up a system to support intake procedures.

Racial, Ethnic, and Religious Issues in Home Health Care

Throughout all phases of home health care service provision, it is essential that the practitioner remain cognizant of racial, ethnic, and religious differences and the resultant issues that may arise. Concern for such matters needs to begin at the point of initial contact.

During the initial exchanges with the client, it might be wise to explore client expectations regarding his or her potential home health care worker. It is not uncommon to have workers who do not reflect the racial, ethnic, or religious backgrounds of the client population. This does not mean that the match will not work. It is necessary to provide cultural orientation to home care service providers and to discuss openly with clients the concerns or, perhaps, biases that they may harbor. Although results may not rival those of the United Nations, if approached properly, a worker and client of different backgrounds can certainly prove to be an excellent fit.

The practitioner's role might include suggesting or initiating training and "sensitivity heightening" sessions for all staff. In addition, those who provide the daily in-home services would benefit from additional information on such things as dietary considerations, rituals, and customs that might affect routine service provision. Discussions with clients during intake and routine visits should always include an opening for clients to express, in a private one-to-one setting, their concerns stemming from racial, ethnic, and other differences. The client must be reassured that there will be no negative repercussions from honest discourse on the topic. Should all these efforts fail, the practitioner must serve as mediator/facilitator in group counseling sessions and, perhaps, ultimately seek out a different client-worker match.

The potential for racial, ethnic, and religious issues to impact the home health care environment goes well beyond the home care worker-client relationship. In taking a history and conducting a psychosocial assessment (see Chapter 6), it is critical that the practitioner bring his or her biases or preconceived ideas to the fore. While it may not be possible to do away with them in an instant, it is certainly possible, and necessary, to keep them clearly in view. Thus when Mrs. Bouvier states that her parents put her on a boat alone when she was 12 years old to send her to work in the United States, record the data objectivity. In addition, it would be unfair to indicate in an assessment that Mrs. B. was abandoned or neglected, for example. Put the facts in a cultural and historical perspective. Was her native country at war at the time? Did her family live in severely substandard conditions in their homeland? Was a girl of 12 considered a woman in the environment from which she came?

The Intake Form

Intake forms can vary greatly according to the specific eligibility criteria established by the agency, but all agencies should have such a tool to both gather and maintain home care information. A formal intake protocol promotes the collection of service data in a standardized and consistent manner for the agency record.

Outside factors that impact on intake form design include the requirements of funding sources and government mandate. In those instances where the funding source requires the use of a specific form, the agency may create a supplemental form to gather additional data deemed important. Although it is necessary to collect a certain amount of information for both eligibility determination and service provision, the collection of extraneous data should be avoided. Keep in mind that an unnecessarily lengthy survey may extend beyond the older person's attention span or may be physically stressful. Overly complex intake tools may even upset the applicants to the point that they determine the service is not worth the indignity or the effort of completing the application.

Certain data should be included in all intake forms for home health care. These include:

- Client name
- Client address
- Client telephone
- Client social security number (this is the commonly accepted form of identification for all social service agencies and government bodies)
- Date of birth
- Financial history (if there is a financial eligibility criterion to satisfy)
- Presenting problem or precipitating event
- Health data—medical history, medications, primary care physician or medical clinic, current diagnosis)
- Governmental benefits
- Emergency contact's name, address, and telephone
- Referral source
- Functional capacity (capacity to perform activities of daily living) to determine degree of care necessary
- Mental capacity
- Language(s)
- Dietary restrictions and allergies
- Informal supports
- Other involved agencies
- Marital status
- Living arrangements (rental, private home, cooperative, condominium, and whether alone or with others)

If there are other agency eligibility criteria (e.g., citizenship, veteran status, etc.), then such questions should naturally be included. A series of sample intake forms may be found in the Appendix.

Confidentiality

It is important to remember that the information collected at intake is confidential and may only be viewed by the involved agency staff, the client, and, in some cases, must be made available to the funding source when requested. Because the sharing of such personal information can be very trying for the service applicant, it is important to inform him or her prior to commencement of questioning that confidentiality is respected. Confidentiality also means that the information to which you are privy should not be shared with others outside of the agency, and conversation regarding clients between agency staff should not take place where others may overhear.

The Initial Home Visit

The fact that an individual has made the effort to initiate and complete the intake/screening process for home care service is indicative of his or her sense of need and willingness to accept assistance. This step is frequently taken in a moment of despair or crisis, a temporary state. As a result, there may be a tendency for the potential client not to pursue service beyond this stage, perhaps electing not to schedule a first home visit. To ensure that the client is given adequate encouragement to access service if he or she so desires, it is highly advisable to set a date for the first home visit at the conclusion of the intake process. Ideally, the first appointment should take place no later than one week to 10 days following intake to guarantee a sense of continuity and concern for the applicant's welfare and needs.

The purpose of the first visit, to conduct a needs assessment, is addressed in the following chapter, but there are some important points to consider when planning the appointment and handling the mechanics of the initial visit:

1. Schedule the first home visit at the end of conducting the intake procedure.
2. Make every attempt to select a mutually agreeable time.
3. Give the client a large-print written reminder of the date.
4. Call the client prior to visiting to remind him or her of who you are, why you are coming, and when.
5. Clearly identify yourself as you attempt to gain access to the client's home.
6. Be respectful of the fact that you are in someone else's home and abide by his or her decisions such as where to sit to conduct the business at hand.
7. Clarify the intended length of the visit before you commence.
8. Upon leaving, give the client your name and telephone number in writing and advise him or her as to the next step in service provision.

Although the focus here is on the client's perspective, it is important not to lose sight of the issue of worker safety. Because clients do not always reside in safe neighborhoods, staff should be aware and take proper precautions. It is not at all inappropriate to request an escort if deemed necessary.

6

Needs Assessment

This chapter addresses the purpose and function of the home health care agency client assessment, including its classic components. Particular attention will be given to the importance of obtaining multiple measures of client status, the advantages and disadvantages of using existing instrumentation that assess older adult need, and the proper treatment of client data once obtained. The distinction between gauging a client's strength as compared to his or her deficits will also be considered.

Once the client's eligibility and appropriateness for home health care has been determined, a thorough assessment of need is performed. Depending on the home health care agency, the assessment of need may be conducted at the point of intake and screening or subsequent to it in a separate interview session. Because the needs assessment is usually rather time consuming, however, entailing a comprehensive gathering of data on the older person's status, it is not likely to be carried out before eligibility for service has been ascertained.

The needs assessment serves the purpose of securing information that will enable the geriatric practitioner to make informed decisions about designing the care plan. A systematic process of information gathering increases the likelihood of an accurate diagnosis and treatment plan. In general, needs assessments serve the function of identifying those conditions evidenced in the older person that require remediation. As indicated in the previous chapter, information is gathered from a variety of sources in gaining an understanding of the older person's situation, including the client, his or her relatives and other informal supports, and health and social service professionals who are acquainted with the individual.

Functional Assessment

At the core of any needs assessment is a desire to obtain a thorough picture of the person's functional status (i.e., an understanding of what the person is and is not able to do). An accurate determination of functional status is ascertained by securing information that reflects client capacity across a range of dimensions including physical and mental/emotional health, social/familial health, economic health, environmental health, and the person's capacity to perform a variety of activities of daily living (ADL). While the geriatric practitioner is certainly capable of administering the average assessment package in its entirety, its multidimensional nature will ensure that the concerns of a variety of professional disciplines will be attended to during the interview, including nursing, social work, medicine, occupational and physical therapy, pharmacy, and the like.

Regardless of the specific aspect of functional status that is being assessed, the home health care practitioner should never lose sight of the position the older person occupies in his or her environment. This assessment of the "person-in-situation" helps to ensure that each individual will be considered in the personal and unique context of his or her own world and support system. Such a perspective enables the practitioner to recognize the possibility that the same infirmity (e.g., a hip fracture or a stroke) can have significantly different implications in terms of need depending on the integrity of person's informal support network, emotional health, housing arrangements, and so on. Put differently, it is imperative to collect information that provides a picture of both the older person's exogenous (external) world and his or her endogenous (internal) world. Any assessment tool that has a particularly strong orientation in one direction or another should be treated with extreme caution (Silverstone, 1981). And, in the final analysis, the clinical judgment of the professional geriatric practitioner should overrule or at least figure strongly in the interpretation of a numerical score obtained from any formal assessment tool (Martin, Morycz, McDowell, Snustad, & Karpf, 1985). Clinical judgment and careful psychosocial scrutiny by the practitioner may particularly come into play when a client takes issue with findings or conclusions derived from an assessment tool.

Ultimately the worker aims to obtain a complete or holistic view of the individual's situation. The responsible practitioner will attempt to identify problem or need areas that impinge on the client's total life sphere. Of course only a limited number of needs may be treatable within the interventive boundaries of a particular home care agency. In such cases the practitioner bears the responsibility of steering the older person to alternative service providers in the community.

Assessment Tools and Packages

During the past 15 years a multitude of assessment tools have been developed (Kane & Kane, 1981). As a result, there is a good chance that a particular package or a modified version of an existing instrument will satisfy the requirements of the typical home health care agency. Because of the easy availability of reliable and valid assessment packages, most agencies do not spend time and energy constructing their own tool. Remember, however, that the trend has been toward more inclusive assessment tools, which has resulted in instruments that some practitioners feel are too time consuming and inflexible, and underscore present performance and capacity at the expense of potential performance. Even so, the advantages of using a structured, formal assessment package (whether it be an already existing tool or your agency's own) are difficult to deny.

The advantages of using previously published assessment packages include the availability of a baseline for comparison and the opportunity eventually to compare your agency's experience in working with older adults with that of other programs that are using identical or similar instrumentation. Existing packages also have a "track record," many having been already tested for validity and reliability. Of course, using an existing tool will save your agency significant time and money in terms of development and testing. On the other hand, an assessment package that is developed in-house will be hand tailored to your own needs and service population. Frequently a good compromise is the middle of the road approach in which you utilize a combination of your own assessment probes and those developed by others (properly cited, of course). In such cases you will still have the opportunity to do some comparative analyses of your service experience and that of other agencies. The instrument you ultimately use should only ask questions about those needs of the client that you can respond to either through your own agency's intervention or by means of a referral to another agency and guard against an assessment process that is inordinately long and, thus, burdensome to a functionally incapacitated older person. In some cases it will be possible to use shortened versions of previously developed assessment packages although the authors of certain tools advise against this.

It is worth mentioning that you should be careful not to jump to false conclusions when using existing assessment tools simply because your client may vary considerably from the preestablished baseline. You will need to take into consideration what may be the special characteristics of the client population you are serving and all dimensions of a person's functional capacity. For example, if your client's score is at the extreme end on one dimension (e.g., physical health) because he or she has a number of identifiable diseases or ailments, you may be quick to jump to the conclusion that he or she is severely dependent. Yet this person may have a great capacity to compensate in other areas of his or her life. Once again, it needs to be emphasized that performing a total assessment is crucial. Responsible and cautious assessments that are performed at periodic points in the service-delivery sequence guard against premature or inaccurate conclusions as to an individual's capacity and frequently fluctuating level of need.

The consequences of misuse of assessment tools is demonstrated in the case of Mr. Fong, a 78-year-old widower:

> Mr. Fong was referred to the local home health care agency by a concerned neighbor who noted both his functional limitations and lack of formal and informal supports. In response to the referral, the agency sent out a worker to perform a multidimensional assessment as an evaluative tool. The resulting scores indicated that Mr. Fong had significant cognitive impairment including disorientation to time and place.
>
> In the hands of an inexperienced practitioner, these scores might have resulted in a referral for supportive in-home care, without further evaluation. Mr. Fong's case practitioner recognized, however, that the assessment results were incongruent with the information provided by the neighbor: that Mr. Fong had been living independently and

without incident for over a year, despite his limitations. Further review
of the case, including a comprehensive physical exam, revealed that
Mr. Fong had been suffering from a stomach ailment for several weeks,
drastically limiting his nutritional intake and causing persistent dehy-
dration. His ill-health was found to be the primary cause of the
apparent confusion. The case plan included the appropriate medical
intervention as well as long-term assistance with ADLs.

Typically, available instruments aim to be multidimensional, comprehensive, and rely on a combination of question-and-answer and
observational formats. A thorough assessment procedure should
measure both objective and subjective need; that is, it should measure the individual's subjective experience or perception of need
along various dimensions as well as the objective reality of his or
her circumstances. For example, the assessment might include a
question as to level of monthly income as well as an indication from
the older person as to how well he or she is managing on his or her
current assets. By objective standards the person may be living an
impoverished life, but he or she does not find this to be disturbing
or immobilizing.

The assessment instrument you ultimately decide to use should
satisfy several criteria (Kane, 1985). These include being: (a) reliable
(in the absence of chance, repeated assessments should yield the
same results); (b) valid (it should have the capacity to measure what
it claims to measure); (c) practical (it should be comfortable for the
practitioner to administer and the client to undergo); and (d) suited
to the client population you serve (i.e., functionally impaired elders
living in noninstitutional settings). Of course, in some circumstances, agencies use specific tools or specific categories of information in order to comply with state regulations that are many times
used to determine eligibility for certain levels of care.

Comprehensive assessments usually take about 45 minutes to one
hour to complete. Kane (1987) has summarized the typical measures
comprising the various components of the clinical assessment.

Physical and cognitive functioning can be measured by such items as:

- Diagnosis
- Symptoms
- Self-reported health, pain, or discomfort
- Days spent in bed during a specified period

- Use of hospitals and/or physicians during a specified period
- Use of medications
- Orientation to time, person, and place
- Extent of short- and long-term memory

Mental/emotional functioning can be assessed in terms of:

- Severity of depression, anxiety, loneliness, emotional well-being, satisfaction with life
- History of psychiatric disorder
- Alcohol and drug dependency

Social functioning is typically measured by assessing:

- Frequency and nature of contacts with family, friends, neighbors, and confidants
- Frequency and nature of social activities, group memberships, and church/synagogue affiliation

ADL functioning is determined by the older person's capacity to:

- Perform self-care activities such as bathing, grooming, eating, dressing, and getting in and out of bed
- Maneuver stairs
- Clean the house and do the laundry
- Cook meals
- Use the telephone
- Pay bills and/or write letters
- Do the shopping

Additional questions may consider the quality of the housing stock and the community in which the older person resides, the adequacy of income and savings, and the current range of community services being received.

Examples of existing comprehensive assessment packages include:

1. The OARS (Older Americans Research and Services) multidimensional functional assessment questionnaire that gathers information on the overall functional status of persons 18 years and older (Duke University, 1978). This instrument has been shown to be valid

and reliable. The OARS questionnaire measures functional status in five areas: physical health, mental health, social health, economic health, and activities of daily living. It also includes a section that measures the extent to which community services are needed and used. The questionnaire takes about 45 minutes to complete. Alternative strategies for examining and scoring the information are available (Fillenbaum, 1987). It is generally recommended that the OARS be used in its entirety. Further information on the OARS questionnaire is available from OARS, Center for the Study of Aging and Human Development, Duke University Medical Center, Durham, NC 27710.

2. The CARE methodology (Gurland & Wilder, 1984) offers a variety of statistically valid and reliable indices that can be combined in hand-tailored fashion to meet the needs of particular community assessment programs. The CARE package incorporates measures of ADL, physical health, mental health, social resources, environmental matters, caregiver strain, economic status, nutrition, and service use. This questionnaire tends to have a psychiatric emphasis.

3. The Multilevel Assessment Inventory (MAI) developed by Lawton, Ward, and Yaffe (1982) at the Philadelphia Geriatric Center has also been shown to be statistically valid and reliable. Like the CARE, MAI allows the user to administer several versions of the questionnaire depending on the capacity of the client and the amount of time available for the assessment process. The MAI has indices that measure ADL, physical health, mental health, social resources, economic status, environmental factors, and client use of time.

Special Tips in Conducting Client Assessments

This section offers a series of special tips and considerations when conducting client assessments. First, it is particularly important for the assessment to include some inquiry into the person's history of falling. It has been determined that clients at high risk of falling tend in particular to pride themselves on their previous autonomy and wish to stay independent at any cost. They may be preoccupied with a life crisis, they may tend not to seek help, and they may believe falls to be inevitable. Persons with assistive devices that help coordination and redistribution of weight are probably less at risk than are alert clients in wheelchairs who are mobile. (Barbieri, 1983).

Second, the assessment of emotional and behavioral problems is often as important as the determination of physical limitation in the client. Psychological and behavioral problems may represent a major source of tension and frustration for the older person as well as for his or her family and friends (Fortinsky, Granger, & Seltzer, 1981). Behavioral status is frequently an extremely useful indicator in predicting how well the person will ultimately deal with physical incapacity. Neglecting self-care and restlessness are among the most frequently reported behavioral problems, while asking repetitive questions, losing things, and forgetting what day it is are common memory problems (Zarit, Reever, & Bach-Peterson, 1980).

Third, be prepared for possible cultural differences in the way older adults cope with functional incapacity. Acceptable behavior in one culture may be unacceptable in another. Don't allow your own cultural biases to influence your assessment of client need. Similarly, differences can be expected to surface in the way older men and women express need. Women have been found more likely get help with the basic activities of daily living (e.g., assistance with walking, dressing, bathing, eating, and grooming) while men are more likely to be assisted with instrumental needs (e.g., assistance with housekeeping, transportation, food preparation, grocery shopping, personal business affairs) (Branch & Jette, 1983).

Fourth, practitioners should be mindful of the potentiality for elder abuse among the clients they serve. The occurrence of elder abuse continues to be underreported, and in most cases action is not taken until the problem reaches crisis proportions. Abuse may surface in the form of neglect, abandonment, malnutrition and starvation, confinement, undermedication and overmedication, withholding of personal and medical care, beating, sexual abuse, and more subtle psychological abuse causing fear (Kinderknecht, 1986). During the course of the assessment the practitioner should be particularly sensitive to the client's comfort level with his or her caretaker, the location and quality of the client's room, and the role that the client's personality and behavior may play in this respect (Kinderknecht, 1986). Conducting confidential interviews with the client and the caretaker may be indicated as part of the comprehensive assessment if abuse is suspected.

Social Supports

Do not underestimate the crucial influence that social supports play in the lives of older persons. Social support, while usually provided by family members, should be conceived of in broad terms. Informal assistance may be available not only from family members, but also from friends, neighbors, clergy, local merchants, and so on. Such persons have traditionally been the predominant providers of socialization and help with personal development, daily living tasks, and personal help during crisis or illness (Cantor, 1985).

A sensitive assessment is able to gauge the strength of all such social supports and, in turn, guard against the possibility of agency home health care assuming a substitutive rather than a supplementary function in relation to the help provided by others. In addition, the assessment process should be sensitive to the possible negative effects that relatives, friends, and others may have on the client's health and, ultimately, the care plan that is established between the older person and the home health care agency (Kaye, 1985b). The presence of social support does not mean it is positive. The extent to which social ties prove to be useful or damaging for the elderly person's well-being depends to a large extent on whom the connections are with and the quality of the interaction rather than the quantity or frequency of contact (O'Brien & Wagner, 1980). The assessment should also include one or more questions that measure the level of stress and strain being experienced by the person's informal caregivers and thus help assess the risk of potential "burnout" on the part of these persons.

Identifying Client Strengths

Because the underlying purpose of the assessment process is to measure or identify deficits, there is likely to be a tendency for service providers to come to see clients as the sum total of their deficits or impairments. It is very important to remember that individuals should ultimately be viewed as the sum total of their strengths. The very fact that a man or woman in his or her late seventies, suffering from multiple disabilities, has survived to the point of seeking help confirms his or her substantial capacity and tenacity. Worker perceptions should, therefore, not be unduly biased during the course of the assessment process. Similarly, an older person who may suffer from considerable physical disability and be restricted in his or her ADLs should not be necessarily assumed to be psychologically frail.

A well-formulated needs assessment can measure an individual's level of wellness or capacity as effectively as it measures a person's need for assistance. And, just as it is crucial to recognize the older person's strengths and capacities during the stage of service delivery (see Chapter 8), it may well be indicated to do the same during the assessment of need.

In the final analysis it should be remembered that the elderly are no different from younger people in certain major respects. The majority are not disabled or dependent; they are not psychologically frail and can, therefore, be dealt with realistically and, when necessary, in a confrontational manner; they have the capacity to learn and thus the potential to solve their own problems. Home health care workers will benefit from periodically reminding themselves that the elderly have been living a long time and have much experience at decision making (Beland, 1984). Their capacity for decision making is likely to be rationally based, including the decision to leave or remain at home when their health and security is threatened.

A closing note is warranted regarding the treatment of information that has been collected by means of the clinical assessment. By definition these data are personal and sensitive and should be treated accordingly. Clients should be advised of the manner in which the information collected during the assessment will be handled and for what purposes it will be used (e.g., preparing the care plan). All such material should be treated with strictest confidentiality.

7

Case Planning

Once adequate information on the status of the elder client has been obtained, case planning can commence. Development of a successful case plan is contingent upon the careful review of accurate clinical assessment data which, in turn, leads to a determination of the type and severity of problems or needs that exist for the older adult and, subsequently, an interventive plan. Case planning is enhanced by collecting assessment information according to a routine format as described in the previous chapter (Kane, 1985). Furthermore, case plans are best constructed within the context of a cooperative and trusting relationship that is established between elder consumers, informal supports, and providers of home health care services. The process of case planning is completed when the practitioner succeeds in translating realistic client needs and wishes into one or more therapeutic interventions offered by the home health care agency in combination with assistance from other human service programs.

This chapter will review a series of techniques for establishing successful case contracts. The critical components of the home health care contract will also be delineated as well as the process whereby a contract is arrived at. Finally, attention will be directed at strategies for motivating elder clients and their informal supports to carry out the plan of care.

Establishing the Contract

Successful home care case plans are not arrived at by chance. They result from a disciplined and thoughtful process that is orchestrated by the geriatric practitioner in consultation with the home health care team and that takes into consideration the preferences of the older person and significant individuals in the elder's life. Case planning that foregoes a rational and systematic effort on the part of the practitioner can lead to serious consequences usually resulting from the absence of mutual contracting and, consequently, a lack of fit or match between specific services and client/family needs and expectations. Grossly inaccurate perceptions of service can easily arise, including the following:

1. Elder clients may harbor unrealistic standards with regard to the performance of home health care staff;
2. Relatives and friends of the client may be confused about their role and function in the home care plan;
3. The older person may assume that the home care staff will perform tasks that are different from those comprising their job descriptions (e.g., scrubbing walls and floors even though heavy cleaning is not part of their responsibility);
4. The older person may expect staff to provide companionship beyond their normal working hours; and
5. Older persons may automatically assume that home care staff will be similar to themselves in terms of their age as well as their racial, ethnic, and cultural backgrounds (Friedman & Kaye, 1979; Kaye, 1985a).

Mutuality of planning is the key to successful case planning. Practitioners are charged with integrating the expressed needs and desires of the client with their own informed judgment and expertise. The most successful case plans are arrived at through mutual discussion rather than agency directive or coercion. Worker coercion will backfire in the long run due to increased likelihood that the older person and/or a relative will lack commitment and, perhaps, be hostile toward or even sabotage the plan once it has been implemented.

Mutuality also means that the expectations of family members will be addressed in the case plan. This requires that active family members be included in the case planning process and in the specification of roles and functions. Their involvement early on will minimize confusion, competition between worker and family members, and feelings of guilt or anger during service delivery. Joint engagement in the contracting sequence ensures that all parties will assume a degree of ownership of the plan and, therefore, responsibility for making it work.

The acceptance of mutual accountability by all parties involved naturally results from a process of mutual planning. That is, the practitioner aims to guarantee that all parties entering into the contract will bear responsibility for respecting and abiding by the plan of action as well as participating in a periodic review of the plan to ensure its continuing appropriateness and integrity.

In addition to mutual planning, the establishment of trust, the building of a relationship, and the promotion of clear communications are pivotal to the construction of the successful case plan. Use of counseling expertise on the part of the geriatric practitioner may be required in order to assure that these processes are adequately attended to (see Chapter 8).

Practitioners who are responsible for case planning and contract development must have an excellent working knowledge of the range of alternative services and products offered by their home health care agency including the cost of care, the frequency and duration of help available, and the profiles of the staff who provide in-home care. In addition, case planning requires a clear understanding of services and programs that are available through other home care programs and related community service agencies. Home care contracts may entail plans to deliver a variety of services including: home-delivered meals; telephone reassurance; friendly visiting; escort; homemaker, home health aide, and home attendant services; counseling; and nursing, medical, dental, and psychiatric services. In addition, case planning may well entail discussions of future service needs that are not home delivered, including adult day care, foster care, congregate housing, and nursing home placement.

Regardless of the quality of planning that goes into the case plan, the final product is likely to reflect less than the optimal set of interventive options given the limitations of resources and alternatives available to the older adult. The case plan, therefore, represents, more or less, a balanced compromise between what is needed and what is available. (For example, an elderly shut-in may optimally need companionship and assistance 7 days a week, but the local home health care program can only provide home attendant services Monday through Friday.)

Components of the Home Care Contract

Successful home care contracts are composed of a series of essential components. The hallmark of a good contract is one in which the components are made explicit to the older adult and informal supports. Communicating the agreement with clarity both verbally and in writing is strongly recommended. Key components of the contract are outlined below:

1. *Specification of Goals and Objectives.* The home care contract should delineate one or more goals and interim objectives of the case plan. The goal of the contract may be as simple as the delivery of a service such as homemaking assistance or more complex such as the expectation that the client will become more active, functioning more fully in daily life activities. A series of progressive interim objectives may be developed in the latter case that could include having the homemaker prepare well-balanced meals, which will result in improved nutritional intake by the client, obtaining a walker to assist the client with ambulation, having the homemaker assist the client in getting to the local park bench to sit for 45 minutes each day, and ultimately enabling the client to be assisted to the corner grocery store for light shopping.

2. *Placement in a Temporal Context.* The plan of care needs to be placed in the context of a time frame. The contract should specify how frequently service will be provided (the number of days each week and hours per day) and for how long a period of time (days, weeks, or months). The plan may specify an absolute time limit based on agency policy or as a result of the requirements of an insurance policy for reimbursement of coverage. Alternatively, the provider and the consumer of home health care services may formally agree to reassess the situation after a certain period of time. Such an agreement should be written into the case plan. It is wise to specify time frames for the achievement of interim or intermediate objectives as well as for the achievement of a plan's final objectives.

3. *Delineation of Payment Schedules.* The contract should include a detailed breakdown of the cost of care. Referred to here is the specification of a schedule of payments, any expectations for contributions on the part of the client, and a determination of whether billing will be made to a third party. If there is to be no fee for the service, this, too, should be made explicit.

4. *Clarification of Roles and Responsibilities.* Essential to contracting is a precise detailing of the respective roles of all parties involved. The contract should specify the responsibilities and functional tasks to be performed not only by home care staff but also by involved relatives as well as the elder client. Appropriate tasks and behaviors for each party to the contract should be outlined. For example, the plan may specify that a client's son will assume the responsibility for home repair and heavy house cleaning, while the homemaker will do the shopping and prepare the lunch time meal. Both will, on the other hand, be available for companionship and providing emotional support on an as-needed basis.

By definition, this part of the contract will specify the range of services or types of assistance that will be provided by the home health care agency. It should also include some indication of those services or types of assistance that are not to be expected of agency staff.

Personal care in the home is steeped in emotionality. If the role and function of in-home staff, relatives, and the older person are unclear, poorly formulated, or misunderstood, problems during the course of service delivery are likely to surface. The passive client may be embarrassed to ask for assistance in perfectly appropriate areas (e.g., help with personal hygiene if incontinent) while the aggressive client will assume that agency staff should perform tasks that extend beyond their job performance profiles (e.g., doing major home repairs or repeatedly running errands). A clear contract specifies the limits of appropriate behaviors for all parties involved including the roles, function, and tasks of significant others.

5. *Achievement of Clarity but not Irrevocability.* Home care contracts are not irrevocable. The older person should know that the plan of care can be changed or modified within certain limits and at any time during the course of service delivery. Because client status is going to change over time, the contract should specify a plan for reassessment and the scheduling of that procedure. Clients need to

understand in no uncertain terms that they have power and control over the plan and ultimately the right to terminate service or ask for a referral to another agency.

Additional Case Planning Recommendations

Armed with client assessment information, the geriatric practitioner should initially attempt to provide the elder with a menu of alternatives. Such a menu may well represent a constellation of potential interventions offered by the practitioner's agency and/or other community programs. The offering of choice has therapeutic value in that it emphasizes the fact that functionally impaired older adults still can retain some degree of control over their own lives. Discussion of alternatives is a morale booster as well and can serve to help stabilize the health status of the older adult (Garner & Mercer, 1982; Hodgson & Quinn, 1980).

The responsible practitioner will realize that it is not his or her job to promote his or her own agency's services only. Rather, he or she needs to be willing to identify the most appropriate service for the client regardless of the source. This obligation will, at times, be difficult to adhere to, but it centers precisely around a professional responsibility to remain accountable to the client. For example, your agency may be limited to the provision of social work, nursing, and home health aide services. Yet during case planning it becomes evident that the older person will benefit most from attending an adult day care program three times a week combined with daily participation in a meals-on-wheels project. Your choice is a clear one: referral of that person to the local community adult day care project and home- delivered meals service.

The initial presentation of a menu of service alternatives to the client should reflect a broad spectrum of available types of assistance. The practitioner and all relevant individuals in the contract development process should then proceed to hone down the alternatives package to a more manageable and realistic set of services for that person. Criteria governing the consideration of alternatives include the client's personal preferences, the external assessment of need, service cost comparisons, and the quality and quantity of available assistance (Lawton, 1978). Figure 7.1 summarizes the advantages and disadvantages that are generally associated with the more common services for functionally impaired older adults.

The successful narrowing of alternatives may require that the practitioner help the client confront strengths and weaknesses. Some clients overemphasize their weaknesses while others remain resolutely stoic and minimize their need for help. There may well be a need to counsel those clients who take either of these unrealistic positions in the hopes that they can be helped to arrive willingly at a more accurate view of their needs. Clinical skills will be called into play at these times (see Chapter 8).

Sometimes the practitioner will need to assume the role of moderator during case planning. In such cases, where there is disagreement between clients and relatives as to the appropriate course of action, the practitioner aims to facilitate constructive discussion by identifying realistic and unrealistic or inappropriate service options.

It should be noted that during times of crisis the process of narrowing alternatives through open discussion will need to be temporarily put off. In these instances (e.g., an unexpected and disabling accident or a sudden and severe stroke) the practitioner will need to determine quickly, without extensive discussion, what type of plan needs to be implemented. In such a situation the case plan will need to be more systematically discussed by all relevant parties at a later point in time when the crisis has passed.

Motivating the Client to Carry Out the Plan of Care

A well-conceived and mutually developed contract is the best insurance that your clients and their families will be motivated to abide by the case plan. Such a plan will not have been imposed on anyone. Client and family members alike will feel they have a stake in that contract because they were responsible for its development.

There are cases, however, in which clients are not realistic and, therefore, may not be satisfied with the plan of care. For example, Mr. Jones, an extremely dependent widower, may feel he is not receiving adequate levels of assistance in performing certain personal activities of daily living, including dressing and grooming. The case plan calls for him to gradually assume increased responsibility in these two areas as he recovers from a minor sprained ankle. In this case the client's position is at odds with the case plan.

Advantages	*Disadvantages*

Community Congregate Housing

Advantages	Disadvantages
Congenial home environment	Requires relatively high level of cognitive and physical functioning
Personal autonomy remains intact	May require relocation from former neighborhood and supports
Some supports available	Limited availability
Age segregation has positive impact	
Possibility of informal reciprocity	
Independent life-style enhances morale and motivation	
Self-care is promoted	
Provides opportunities for interaction	

Foster Families

Advantages	Disadvantages
All functional levels are appropriate	Limited availability
Provides home environment and "surrogate family"	Not appropriate for drug or alcohol addicts, wanderers, or violent persons
Provides opportunities for interaction and affection	
Client is matched with family to facilitate success	
High level of care is possible	
Improvement in functioning is possible	

Adult Day Care

Advantages	Disadvantages
Provides opportunity for meaningful activity	Transportation is required
Often a physician is available for consultation	Limited medical facilities and capabilities
Provides opportunity for socialization and interaction	Could cost as much as or more than a nursing home
Provides respite for caregiver	Many day care centers do not accept very demented clients
Enriches interactional skills enabling clients to relate better to families and caregivers	
Promotes sense of control	
Gives sense of belonging and identification with people who care	
Provides structured environment responsive to needs	
Can accommodate the frail and disabled as well as the emotionally or medically unstable	
Restores self-esteem by establishing new roles	
Age peer support groups can have positive impact	
Promotes exercise of autonomy and assertiveness in a safe environment	

Figure 7.1. Advantages and Disadvantages of Common Geriatric Services

Advantages   *Disadvantages*

Day-Care Hospital

Permits comprehensive assessment
of health state and needs

Valuable to get out of the house
regularly

Physician able to provide continuing
care without hospitalization

Enables patient in the hospital to
return home quicker by providing
continued support while patient
readjusts to independent living

Prevents or postpones institutionalization

Incorporates many therapeutic/
rehabilitative features including:

- medical consultation
- speech therapy
- physical therapy
- occupational therapy
- personal care and hygiene training
- nutritional counseling
- activity programs
- nursing procedures (bathing,
  attendance to medication, bowel
  and bladder care)
- hot-cooked meal

Inappropriate for Alzheimer's disease
victims

Transportation tends to be required

Nursing Home

Around-the-clock supervision

Around-the-clock-access to
nursing staff

Reimbursement from Medicare/
Medicaid

Opportunity to interact with
age peers

Sheltered environment

Available to people at all levels
of need

Provides a home to people whose
condition requires more care than
they or family members are able
to give

Loss of control over many aspects of life

Loss of previous home

Promotes chronic dependency

Clients become less able to leave as
time passes

Custodial rather than rehabilitative

Loss of independence

Loss of privacy

Potentially damaging to health

Emphasis on medical, not social, model

Client may not have had a choice to enter
the nursing home, which creates adverse
effects

Figure 7.1. Continued

Advantages	Disadvantages
Home Health Care	
Cost-effective when disability is not severe	Medicare reimbursement inhibits use and often limits home health care to skilled nursing
Contributes to independent life-style	Formal home care can become costly when patient is severely incapacitated
Prevents or postpones institution-alization	
Familiar home environment may enhance client's motivation and response to treatment	
Provides direct care and emotional support	
Client gets high level of care due to interdisciplinary efforts of home health care team	
Includes a wide variety of assistance including:	

- medical care and supervision
- nursing
- social work services
- physical therapy
- occupational therapy
- speech therapy
- inhalation therapy
- medical technician services
- appliance, equipment, and sterile supply services
- nutritional guidance
- transportation for client
- homemaker/home health aide services

Figure 7.1. Continued

How can Mr. Jones be motivated to assume some responsibility for himself? The question is a difficult one to answer; however, the strategy may well be one that focuses on the offering of incentives. The ideal incentive is to activate a process whereby Mr. Jones is counseled so as to understand why a particular service plan is appropriate for him. If, however, an attitudinal change in thinking is not likely to be forthcoming, a behavioral incentive may be needed. For example, it could be explained to Mr. Jones that if he assumes responsibility for shaving and brushing his own hair, then the home health aide will be freed up to prepare lunch. In this case a tradeoff has been arrived at whereby the client is rewarded for responsible behavior with agency assistance in a more demanding area of his daily life.

In their daily practice, geriatric practitioners will normally choose between the two types of motivational strategies outlined above: (a) positive attitudinal change in which the client achieves insight into his or her behavior, and (b) positive behavioral change in which desirable incentives are offered for improved behavior or adherence to the case plan. When all else fails, however, a disincentive can be offered. The strongest disincentive is likely to be the warning that services may need to be withdrawn. This may be appropriate in a situation where the client, by disregarding the case plan, creates a risk for both himself or herself and agency personnel.

For those clients who require motivation, the use of positive reinforcement is always preferable and represents the first avenue of recourse. Even limited progress on the part of the client deserves reward and recognition.

It is useful to remember that it may be strategically wise to enlist the support of active family members and friends in any effort to motivate the elder client. A spouse, son, or daughter may prove helpful in encouraging a change in behavior on the part of the older person. In some cases, however, it is the family member or next door neighbor who needs to be encouraged to respect the case plan because he or she is the impediment (Kaye, 1985b). This is especially likely to be the case when informal supports are family members who are playing out years and years of emotional discord within the context of the plan of care. Inevitably, a good bit of emotional baggage can impact the case plan and ultimately weaken the contract, which has been arrived at between agency, elder, and family.

8

Service Delivery

Service delivery in home health care commences with the implementation of a plan of care contract that has been entered into by the elder client and the service provider. Successful service delivery is, of course, contingent upon a multitude of factors, some over which the agency may have little control. This chapter will consider a series of skill factors considered pivotal in realizing a successful outcome and over which the agency can be expected to exercise some influence. Specifically, we will discuss the central importance of service coordination, quality of care monitoring, team work, the use of crisis intervention techniques, and short-term counseling skills.

Coordination of Services

For any given home care client, your agency may be providing services at the same time that other agencies and informal providers are involved. As a result there is a need for case or service coordination. Often referred to as case management in the human services, this function aims to minimize the occurrence of overlaps and gaps in service delivery. In some instances the absence or duplication of services may not be serious. For example, if chore service is not available one day or if two different agencies are providing telephone reassurance services to the same client, no serious consequences are likely either for the client or the agency. On the other hand the consequences of duplicative or unavailable service may be serious, even life threatening. For instance, when more than one community program is involved in overseeing the administration of medication to a frail person, the accidental doubling or skipping of a dose can have serious, if not life-threatening, consequences. Case management can serve to prevent such occurrences.

Case managers aim to assess client need, connect individuals to services, and then coordinate and monitor the service delivery sequence (Kaye, 1988). In general such services are important given the increasing complexity of service systems in most localities, the absence of standardized services, the short supply of resources to meet human needs, the need for programs to reach the appropriate target population, the state of flux in which many programs find themselves, as well as the hesitancy, ignorance, and mistrust that many older persons have for human service programs (Steinberg, 1985).

Moxley (1989) has defined a case manager as:

> a designated person (or team) who organizes, coordinates, and sustains a network of formal and informal supports and activities designed to optimize the functioning and well-being of people with multiple needs. (p. 17)

By means of these activities, states Moxley (1989), the case manager aims to accomplish the following three central goals:

1. To promote when possible the skills of the client in accessing and utilizing these supports and services,
2. To develop the capacities of social networks and relevant human service providers in promoting the functioning and well-being of the client, and
3. To promote service effectiveness while attempting to have services and supports delivered in the most efficient manner possible. (p. 17)

Moxley (1989) maintains that case managers need to perform five key practice functions if the goals as described above are to be achieved. These functions encompass assessment activities, service planning, the delivery of interventions, monitoring the implementation and accomplishment of the client's service plan, and evaluating the impact of the service delivery plan. This perspective on the case management function is a useful one in the context of home health care. The five practice functions explicated by Moxley should, in fact, be considered crucial to the case practitioner's work in home health care and are addressed repeatedly through this book.

The case manager's role in home health care should include:

1. Maintaining an up-to-date inventory of the client's service providers and services received. Such an inventory must not only be current but detailed as well. For example, knowing that a client receives meals-on-wheels is not enough. The case practitioner must know on which days meals are provided and whether the service is provided on holidays. Exceptions to the normal scheduling of services are not uncommon and essential information for the practitioner performing the case management function. The use of form/flow charts to keep track of what has been done and what needs to be done for the client can serve as a quick means of gathering and reviewing case information.

2. Once the inventory of client services has been taken, the case manager's responsibility becomes one of ensuring that no crucial gaps or overlaps in service exist. This may require active intervention, both with the elder client and one or more service providers, in order that the plan of care be gapfilling and nonduplicative.

3. The practitioner needs to communicate to all other service providers early on that he or she will bear responsibility for the case management role. In similar fashion the elderly client and his or her relatives and significant others need to be advised of who will assume the case management function. Of course the home health care case practitioner may or may not be the appropriate professional to assume the responsibilities of the case manager. That is, such a role should probably not be a self-appointed one. Rather, through discussion with the client, members of the family, and other community service providers, it should be decided which professional is best positioned to assume service coordination duties. Regardless of who eventually assumes the responsibility, it is essential that the function be fulfilled.

4. A responsible case manager will diligently seek feedback from all parties involved in the welfare of the client (family members,

friends, or other service providers) in order to assess how effectively and efficiently the formal and informal network of services is being delivered.

5. Finally, it will be important to conduct ongoing and regular assessments of the adequacy of the total service package because the conditions and needs of home health care clients can change significantly from one day to the next. This reassessment process will lead frequently to the periodic modifications in the overall service delivery package as necessary over time.

Essential skills in successfully performing the case management or service coordination role include organizational management, people management, assessment, and observational expertise. To be a good case manager requires the capacity to reach out for feedback as to the status of the person receiving help. The burden will become quickly an intolerable one if you take it upon yourself to observe all changes in the needs of the client. This is especially the case in home health care given the degree of isolation in which this kind of service is carried out—that is, within the confines of the client's home. The ability to plan well in advance is critical as well (e.g., don't wait until Christmas eve to arrange for home-delivered meals for your client on Christmas and New Year's Day given the fact that so few community programs are likely to offer the service at that time).

Of course, as Bumagin and Hirn (1990) remind us, locating services and knowing their eligibility requirements constitute only a portion of the case manager's responsibility. Of equal importance is being aware of the emotional impact of services on the older person and the consequent necessity in many cases for counseling. In home health care it is not uncommon for the case manager to be responsible for performing certain short-term and crisis-oriented counseling functions as well as the more concrete tasks of service coordination. The counseling function will be addressed later in this chapter.

Case practitioners engaged in the case management function for substantial periods of work time may find one or more of a growing number of specialized publications on the subject to be of help. For example, the *Case Management Advisor*, published by American Health Consultants of Atlanta, Georgia, is a newsletter addressing the specific needs of case management professionals, including such topics as reimbursement, strategies for ensuring quality care, legal issues, ethical questions, new and proposed legislation, clinical treatments, and management of various client groups.

Monitoring Quality of Care

Quality of care monitoring in home health care should be concerned with the goodness of fit between two pivotal components of care: (a) client need, and (b) service attributes. A good fit between the two components suggests good quality of care; a poor fit between the two often translates into poor quality of care. For example, if the case practitioner has assigned a nurses aide to cook meals and provide personal care services for Ms. Anderson, who is actually capable of caring for herself, then the fit between client need and service attributes is poor. The fit is considered poor even though the service being provided is a good one being delivered in a professional and competent manner.

The perspective on quality of care being offered here includes, but goes beyond, traditional views of quality service delivery, which usually entail providing services in a punctual, thorough, and thoughtful manner. This means that case practitioners should continue to monitor the thoroughness and timeliness of chore services being provided by the homemaker or home attendant who has been assigned to the case, but the practitioner must also periodically ensure that client need and service attributes display good fit. Quality of care monitoring is a two-dimensional function that requires close attention at both levels.

Quality of care monitoring is considered to fall within the set of responsibilities of the home health care case manager. Monitoring responsibilities can be adequately carried out in a variety of ways—through periodic home visits, telephone calls to the client, and case conferences with the various providers of home health care services. Formal and informal measures of service satisfaction taken of the client should be performed. The kinds of questions to be asked of the elder client in assessing client satisfaction include:

1. Is the quality of service you are receiving adequate?
2. Are the services being provided meeting your needs?
3. Are you satisfied with the amount of help you are receiving?

4. Are the services you are receiving helping you to deal more effectively with your problems?
5. All things considered, are you satisfied with the services you are receiving?
6. If you were to need help again in the future, would you use our program? Would you recommend our program to a member of your family? To friends?

Case practitioners whose responsibilities encompass quality of care monitoring will need to keep abreast of the most current approaches to home health care service delivery because these are now rapidly changing. For instance, just 15 years ago personal emergency response systems (PERS) were virtually unheard of. These portable, push button, electronic devices that allow help to be summoned 24 hours a day by means of the existing telephone service are now found in the homes of several million older and disabled adults. And there are now at least 20 companies competing in the PERS market with programs now available through a network of thousands of hospitals and health centers throughout the United States (Buglass, 1989).

The miniaturization and increased portability of communication and medical technologies may well alter the very definition of what entails quality home care in the years ahead. Other high-technology medical devices now commonly available in the homes of the functionally impaired include: artificial nutrition and hydration equipment, mechanical ventilation for life support, apnea monitors, platelet infusion devices, morphine drips, computerized health monitoring equipment, bone growth simulators, home dialysis machines, and more. In-home communications technologies include automatic telephone dialing systems such as PERS, in-home computers for medication and nutrition self-instruction, electronic safety systems, and even robotics (Kaye & Reisman, 1991b). It has been projected that it is this segment of the for-profit sector of the medical home care market that will experience the greatest growth in the near-term future (Kane, 1989). Case practitioners who keep abreast of these developments will be able to encourage their older clients to decide early on whether such home care technology will represent an upgrading of the quality of care they receive or an unnecessary add-on that leads to a situation in which excess interventions have intruded into their lives.

Technology importation to the home is bound to raise a range of exceedingly complex ethical concerns for the staff of community home care agencies (Coile, 1990; Macklin & Callahan, 1990). Some case practitioners can expect to be engaged in the development of guidelines for dealing with potential ethical issues or conflicts, to determine approriate staff roles in such cases, to identify the organization's stance on specific ethical issues, and to be available to respond to individual cases as they arise. In this regard home care agencies, in similar fashion to long-term care institutions, may need to consider using ethics committees or similar ruling bodies in addressing issues of medical ethics, life-prolongation technologies, and determination of agency policy (Reamer, 1987). The Hastings Center (1987) maintains that all health care organizations should have explicit policies regarding resusitation as well as formal processes for communicating do-not-resuscitate (DNR) orders between institutions and emergency medical personnel.

Home care clients and their families continue to have little concrete knowledge of their legal rights and responsibilities during the course of service delivery. The fact that the federal Patient Self-Determination Act (PSDA) took effect on December 1, 1991 (Public Law 101-508) served to underscore the evolving legal mandate that home care agencies (as well as hospitals, nursing homes, and hospices) engage in the implementation of a program of education promoting the client's participation in the direct health care decisions affecting his or her life, including an understanding of all advance directives in the state in which they reside. Clients have a right to understand the availability and logistics of do-not-resuscitate (DNR) orders and living wills (now recognized formally in 48 states) as well as their rights regarding access to and refusal of medical technology. Patient education may open a "Pandora's Box" for home care administrators, case practitioners, and other home care staff in this regard, but there appears to be a moral and legal obligation to enlighten consumers (Randall, 1989). Proactive rather than reactive intervention not only benefits clients, but presumably reduces the burden carried by agency personnel as well (Kaye, 1991; Kaye & Reisman, 1991b).

From a regulatory perspective, requirements for maintaining high-quality home care services continue to be quite variable from one program to the next. Quality assurance standards differ depending on the type of funding that is available for services provided (e.g., Medicare, Medicaid, Older Americans Act) and the classification of services offered (homemaker service, home health aide service, visiting nurse service). Establishing hard and fast guidelines for service delivery in home care, as in many fields in the human services, is complex and, at times, inadequate. Until we have succeeded in establishing clear outcome measures of home care services rendered (and this remains difficult), we are more apt to turn to "input" measures of service such as careful selection, training, and supervision of staff than "outcome" measures that gauge the results or products of services rendered (Moore, 1988).

In many cases national standards have been developed (by the National HomeCaring Council for homemakers and home health aides, for example) but are not uniformly followed. The least amount of oversight and regulation for quality assurance appears to have been in the areas of high-technology services (as described above) and homemaker services (Moore, 1988).

Geriatric case practitioners in Medicare-certified home care agencies can expect to find the most developed standards for service delivery and monitoring. The standards in these programs are national rather than state or local. The same set of national standards for quality assurance in Medicare-certified programs are used by Medicaid programs. Quality assurance for Title XX Social Services Block Grant Programs and Older Americans Act Programs require little or no adherence to national standards but, rather, rely on state and local guidelines. Depending on the category of program in which the geriatric case practitioner is employed, voluntary sector standards and accredited status may need to be adhered to. Among the standards-setting organizations currently operating in this capacity are the National HomeCaring Council, the Joint Commission on Accreditation of Healthcare Organizations, the National League for Nursing, the Council on Accreditation of Services for Families and Children, state accrediting programs, and programs operated by national proprietary home care chains such as Upjohn Healthcare Services (Moore, 1988). These accrediting bodies offer various educational materials that may be particularly helpful for home care practitioners engaged in training, education, supervision, and quality assurance. For example, the National HomeCaring Council offers training materials for working with high-tech clients and their families (Nassif, 1987), cancer patients and their families (Nassif, 1986a, 1986b), persons with developmental disabilities (Gilbertson, 1981), and supervision generally (National HomeCaring Council, 1982). These materials are especially geared to practitioners who work with and/ or supervise homemakers and home health aides.

Periodically, federal and state legislation addresses quality assurance issues in home care. In addition to the case practitioner's responsibility for understanding and adhering to any and all quality assurance requirements that apply to a particular home care agency, such an individual will also need to decide whether to assume an advocate's role in promoting improved standards of care in this still evolving field of service.

Regardless of one's formal responsibilities in home care, monitoring quality of care should be integrated into the daily activities of every geriatric case practitioner. Kranz (1989) argues that all home health care programs should have a formal model of quality care monitoring or quality assurance (QA) as defined by the Joint Commission on Accreditation of Healthcare Organizations, which currently accredits home care companies. The Joint Commission's standards entail a 10-step process (Joint Commission on Accreditation of Healthcare Organizations, 1988a; Joint Commission on Accreditation of Healthcare Organizations, 1988b). Kranz (1989) has summarized the steps involved in developing your agency's written plan and design of activities as follows:

1. Assigning responsibility
2. Identifying the scope of care
3. Identifying important aspects of care
4. Developing indicators
5. Determining thresholds
6. Collecting and organizing data
7. Evaluating care when thresholds are reached
8. Taking action to improve care
9. Assessing the effectiveness of actions taken
10. Communicating findings

For the above process to be successful, direct-service staff need to be directly involved in developing the QA plan and the tools used for data collection as they are likely to be the best informed in terms of what are likely to be realistic indicators of service and care performance. QA standards as described by the Commission tend to be medically related and usually fall within the domain of a nurse (e.g., standards of care for congestive heart failure may include patient weight taken at each visit, monitoring blood pressure, pulse and respiration, assessing lung sound, instructing the patient concerning the dose and frequency of medication, assessing lower extremity edema, etc.). The geriatric case practitioner can make an important contribution to the quality of care provided by ensuring that QA plans, in addition to attending to the medical/physical indicators and thresholds of care provided, include adequate attention to social, psychological, and emotional indicators of care as well. Making QA a planned process that benefits from the input of a QA Committee is strongly recommended by the Joint Commission and is commonly expected of Medicare-certified home care agencies (Kranz, 1989).

Working With Other Team Members

The importance of team work in home health care has been spelled out in detail in Chapter 3. Because it can be argued that team work is most critical during the course of service delivery a few points bear repeating.

Regularized contact between all service providers will avoid unnecessary duplication of service. The whole point of a team is that each member has a somewhat different functional role and area of expertise. Different roles need to be recognized and clearly communicated—one staff might perform chore services, one might attend to the medical needs of the client, one member of the team might best attend to particular emotional issues that have surfaced in the older person's life, and still another person might carry supervisory responsibility over the functioning of the team. Clear explication of various staff roles will ensure that service providers do not tread into the functional areas of others (beyond, of course, those instances when some overlap may be expected to occur normally).

Practitioners would do well to be particularly on guard for the possibility of role conflict between nurses and social workers due to possible overlap in these professionals' perceived responsibilities for assessing psychosocial needs and evaluating the mental health status of elder clients (Fessler & Adams, 1985). Task performance conflicts of this type should be dealt with and resolved at the earliest possible point in time. Monitoring such conflict needs to be ongoing and aggressive. Promoting open dialogue between home health care staff may help avert the dynamics that contribute to role conflicts, competition, and eventual disruption of services to clients (Fessler & Adams, 1985). In similar fashion, experience has shown that considerable overlap in function may surface in the work of homemakers and home health aides. Case planners should consider the benefits of utilizing a generic homemaker/home health aide in such instances where it appears the functions of these two staff are inextricably linked for a given case assignment (Lee & Stein, 1980).

Practitioners functioning as team coordinators and case managers should always be aware of the special challenges facing various members of the team. In particular, they need to make those staff who have traditionally held more tenuous team positions (e.g., homemakers/home health aides) to feel they are a vital part of the overall service plan. Concrete recognition of each member's contributions is vital so as to minimize feelings of alienation or nonimportance and to maximize efficiency and job satisfaction (Moore & Layzer, 1983).

It is incumbent that members of the team not lose sight of the fact that the purpose of the team is to provide good quality care for the client. Members must be on guard against becoming embroiled in power struggles, turf issues, and other interpersonal conflicts that in the long run are not beneficial to the client. Clarity of mission—that is, quality service for the client—is pivotal.

Crisis Intervention Techniques

One of the classic definitions of crisis intervention was developed by Howard Parad (1965):

> Crisis intervention means entering into the life situation of an individual, family, or group to alleviate the impact of a crisis inducing stress in order to help mobilize the resources of those directly affected, as well as those who are in the significant "social orbit." (p. 2)

Sherman (1985) maintains that crisis intervention techniques may be particularly useful for work with community-based elderly (such as recipients of home care services). He considers crisis as an upset in a steady state in which previous coping mechanisms are no longer adequate for regaining equilibrium. Crises in elderly home care clients can be brought on by uncontrollable states of anxiety and/or depression (both of which are common conditions in the elderly in general). Common home care crises for which the geriatric case practitioner should be on the lookout for include depressive/anxiety reactions to:

- The death of a spouse, other close relative, or life-long friend
- Downturns in the health status (either physical or mental) of a home-bound client
- Announcements from Medicare, Medicaid, Supplemental Security Income and other entitlement/benefits offices that advise the older person of changes in coverage or procedures
- Overwhelming medical bills for prescription drugs or treatment
- The disruption of a community service (including home care) or changes in the staffing patterns of services being provided

Reactions to each of the above situations may reach crisis proportions in part because of particular anxieties common to the person in later life, including a sense of loss of life defenses, rigid thinking, fear of loneliness, and suspiciousness. In each case noted above, the older adult may interpret the event as another example of his or her increased vulnerability and heightened dependence on the assistance of others such as home care staff. While the examples of precipitating factors outlined above are at first glance very different, each can represent a major loss or threat to the person's well-being and, therefore, result in the need for immediate intervention on the part of the case practitioner.

Crises by definition tend to be time limited—anywhere from 1 to 6 weeks. It is for this reason that rapid intervention and a brief treatment period is essential (Caplan, 1961; Rapoport, 1970).

Practice guidelines for crisis intervention with the elderly include:

1. Helping clients' recognize those factors or events (both explicit and implicit) that have led to a disruption in their functional state. Here both the practitioner and the client need to discuss and agree to what the precipitating event actually was.

2. Mutually arriving at a formulation of the problem that makes possible a restructuring or reordering of the crisis. The event is, in a sense, put into perspective or context such that it is given a "history"

and, therefore, structure. This procedure aims to diminish the irrational characteristics of certain responses and emphasize that it is manageable.

3. Marshalling all available resources to deal with the problem, including the personal resources of the client, one's social support network of family, friends, and neighbors, and formal community resources, including mutual aid and self-help support groups. The use of significant others may be particularly crucial during crises as providers of support (Sherman, 1985).

Good crisis intervention entails encouragement on the part of workers for clients to express openly their feelings of fear and anger and manage their own dysfunctional behavior through the process of ventilation. The practitioner also needs to be reassuring, empathic, and accepting, promoting rational responses to what may at times appear to be irrational behaviors by elderly clients.

For isolated homebound elderly, the temporary disruption of homemaker, home health aide, or chore services can easily precipitate a crisis. Similarly, a service may continue uninterrupted, but turnover in the persons assigned to deliver home care services may prove particularly disturbing, especially if the older client had established a close attachment to the original person. Furthermore, crises may surface during the early phases of home care service because the older person is forced to realize that he or she can no longer function autonomously. The presence of a stranger in the home can also precipitate a crisis.

Of course home care crisis intervention may be appropriately performed by means of rapid, well-planned, concrete actions rather than solely mental health counseling. In fact, home care counseling usually entails the delicate balancing of both emotional and concrete support. Prompt arrangements for substitute services when coverage is unexpectedly interrupted, or preliminary introduction of new workers before they begin their full schedules of work with clients can be extremely helpful in heading off difficult situations before they become full-blown crises:

Mrs. Washington first met her home attendant, Mary, following surgery. The initial case plan, developed in conjunction with Mrs. Washington herself, stipulated that home attendant services would be provided for approximately three weeks. It was anticipated that, by this time, Mrs. Washington would have returned to her former state of independent functioning. Although the client, a proudly independent single woman, was resistant to any help and to having "a stranger" in her home, she was agreeable to this *temporary* intervention. An unanticipated series of medical problems resulted in the permanent full- time assignment of Mary to this case. By this time Mrs. Washington had begun calling Mary her "friend," and the two developed a very close and caring client-worker relationship.

After a year and a half, Mary was preparing to leave the agency and her role as Mrs. Washington's attendant. Mary informed the case practitioner and the two developed a case plan to manage the transition that they knew could precipitate a crisis for the client. Mary herself explained the situation to Mrs. Washington, additional short-term counseling was instituted, and Mary and the case practitioner introduced the new attendant to Mrs. Washington to emphasize continuity of care.

Short-Term Counseling Skills

In work with the elderly it is not uncommon for concrete services to be offered in combination with counseling services. Counseling provided through home health care programs is more likely to be short-term-oriented rather than ongoing. It will also more likely be task centered rather than psychotherapeutically focused. Issues of major concern in counseling with the elderly entail chronic illness and disability, death, and dying, the awareness of physical disorders, adjusting to limitations, understanding specific diseases, complying with prescribed procedures, grieving for the loss of others, ethnicity and aging, love, marriage and sexuality (Knight, 1986).

The initial phase of elder counseling focuses on the importance of active listening, the setting of congruent goals, and the establishment of a mutually agreeable contract (Bumagin & Hirn, 1990). These activities are, of course, the same skills and techniques central to successful home care intake and screening (see Chapter 5), assessment (see Chapter 6), and case planning (see Chapter 7).

As short-term counseling proceeds, the case practitioner should be prepared to deal with possible resistance on the part of the older person. Dealing with issues of loss in the areas of health, family supports, finances, and so on are extremely difficult. In addition, simple solutions are not likely to be forthcoming. Resistance may surface in the form of disappointment, frustration, discouragement, and ambivalence on the part of the older person. Inordinate numbers of canceled or forgotten appointments, undue anger directed toward the case practitioner or other home care staff, and inordinate fear expressed by the client toward members of his or her family may all signal feelings of ambivalence and resistance toward problem resolution. In some cases with home care clients, older persons may minimize or deny their incapacities and need for help out of fear that they might no longer be visited by relatives or, worse, be admitted to a home for the aged or nursing home (Bumagin & Hirn, 1990).

Clinical interventions with older adults and their families may be required if one or more persons are expressing intolerable levels of anxiety or tension over the plan of care in the home, the respective responsibilities and tasks of different persons, or fear of the future. Mobilizing the family and encouraging relatives to work positively with each other in the context of the home care situation is frequently at the core of counseling elders and their families. When working with intergenerational families it is important for the practitioner to be able to distinguish between conflict among family members that is acceptable and even healthy and that which is not (Herr & Weakland, 1979). Some elders and their children traditionally argue over such matters as politics, religion, and the like. These "fights for fun" should not be discouraged simply because the older person is experiencing a period of functional decline.

On the other hand, power struggles that have "no clear demarcation of when the fight is over and an unwillingness to stop fighting until there is a clear winner or loser" are potentially destructive power struggles or "fights for blood" (Herr & Weakland, 1979). They need to be carefully monitored by the case practitioner lest they unduly jeopardize the well-being of the older client and serve to sabotage the home care plan of care.

A problem area common to home care counseling is the strained relationship that evolves between family caregivers and older victims of Alzheimer's disease and related disorders. The practitioner should be prepared to direct his or her effort toward helping all parties involved adjust to this devastating disease. This may include dealing with psychological reactions to the disease, improving the conditions in the home environment of the older adult, and reducing or controlling the stress experienced by informal caregivers. Often the difficulty deals with the idea that a parent has become childlike and that a child will need to assume the caretaking or parenting role. Most feelings of stress and demoralization pertain to the expectation of eventual institutionalization and a sense of frustration, futility, and even guilt over the relative's dislike for having taken on the caregiving role. Both the caregiver and care recipient may sense that there is no place to turn for help and no treatment that will help. In part, the burden of what may feel like a "36-hour day" is the lack of knowledge regarding what to expect in terms of changes in the psychological and physical condition of the victim of this disease (Mace & Rabins, 1981). Practitioners can be of great help by informing relatives of the symptomatology to be expected of Alzheimer's disease so inappropriate behavior is not misinterpreted. Accurate information about the diagnosis and prognosis (offered in consultation with the family physician) also appears to help families cope better with the behavioral problems associated with this disease, as well as encourage adaptation to the progressive changes as they emerge, and make more adaptive long-term care plans (Glosser, Wexler, & Balmelli, 1985). Remember, however, that even when physicians are careful to inform families and clients about diagnosis and prognosis, the shock may be such that the information is not fully assimilated. Ongoing communication between physician, family, client, and home care staff should therefore be encouraged.

Practitioners working with Alzheimer's patients should, according to LaBarge (1981), maintain a strong positive regard for the person, and must be empathetic and skilled at perceiving the internal frame of reference of the victim of the disease. Direct eye contact, close observation of all cues, and precise listening is essential. Supportive therapy is likely to be the dominant strategy along with suggestions for structuring the environment so as to encourage easy to follow routines for the older person.

Participation in caregiver support groups can also serve as an important outlet for stress reduction for involved family members, especially as the disease progresses into the later stages (Pratt, Schmall, Wright, & Cleland, 1985; Schmidt & Keys, 1985; Wasow, 1986). Support group participation should be encouraged for men as well as women engaged in caregiving activities. Men may need to be especially encouraged to make use of this community resource because of their reluctance to participate in group programming of this type (Kaye & Applegate, 1990).

Among the techniques that may be used in dealing with elder clients suffering from organic brain syndromes such as Alzheimer's disease is reality orientation. This technique, which is based on neurological theory, maintains that disorientation occurs when brain cell synapses are atrophied or disconnected. Repetitious exercise is focused on with the goal being the reinforcement of former processes and behaviors of the older person. Reality orientation and similar techniques such as remotivation therapy, provide the client with a reality anchor. These techniques tend to depend to a considerable degree on the use of incentives and concepts of reinforcement. Such methods are, however, time consuming and expensive. In addition, of course, they cannot reverse the course of such diseases as Alzheimer's.

Family counseling may also be indicated when members of the family evidence inaccurate views of their role in relations to the role of the home care staff in caring for the older person. Such counseling, which may tend to be task centered, can help prevent duplicative care, conflicting messages, and outright confusion in terms of who should be doing what during the course of service provision.

Tonti (1983) and Tonti and Silverstone (1985) have summarized a series of interventive procedures recommended for clinical intervention with families of the elderly. These are outlined in Figure 8.1. In each case a family system concept is highlighted and the practical interventions to be considered by the professional are noted. As highlighted, the practitioner's role can be an active one in which assistance is provided in educating, clarifying, and promoting open communications between the relevant family members involved.

Among the techniques to be used by the practitioner in moving the therapeutic process forward are feedback and clarification, reflection and hypothesis, exploration, offering alternatives, and confrontation (Bumagin & Hirn, 1990). These are elaborated on briefly below.

Feedback involves restating the older person's words and asking if they were heard accurately. *Clarification* entails a request for additional detail or explanation of a statement made by the older person. *Reflection* and *hypothesis* entail restating the older adult's problem, dissatisfaction, or complaint and offering one or more reasons for it. *Exploration* may be pursued by the worker if the testing of a particular hypothesis appears warranted. Thus the practitioner will request additional description on a particular issue suggested by his

Family System Concept	Aged System	Intervention
(1) Family boundary: Defines the membership of the "family" and marks the relationship between people inside the family.	Time and distance may change the constituency of the family. Nonfamily included, while relatives who are not involved may be excluded.	(a) Extending the boundary —may need to include alienated family or include friends or neighbors in more involved roles with the elder. (b) Strengthening boundaries—creating space between people where over involvement has created problems of burnout, use of respite programs, day care, etc. (c) Clarifying boundaries— by setting up contracts and discussing obligations and commitments of family members to elder and vice versa.
(2) Tasks: The work the family needs to perform.	Dealing with losses, chronic illness, societal pressures.	(a) Identification. (b) Provide information and education about aging tasks. (c) Help prioritize tasks. (d) Help identify blocks to task performance. (e) Restructure tasks as transactional events important for everyone.
(3) Tension level/homeostasis: The level of tension at which the family feels most comfortable and will work to maintain.	Tension may be increased due to fragility of the elder and the anxiety that the frailty creates in the family.	(a) Educating family about process they are involved in. (b) Involving others to relieve tension through support: 1. Home health aides. 2. Social workers. (c) Problem-solving around tension creating issues. (d) Supporting family to make clear choices as to how they wish to care for their elder.

Family System Concept	Aged System	Intervention
(4) Reverberation: Anything that affects one member affects entire system.	Tendency to try to isolate elder from rest of family to reduce and control reverberation.	(a) Make tendency explicit. (b) Speak for elder if necessary. (c) Support reactions of others to elder's statements. (d) Open channels of communication.
(5) Equifinality: There are many ways to change a system.	The elder's losses and frailty often make change through the elder most difficult and least desirable.	(a) Help other family members to change to support elder. (b) Involve other systems. (c) Change other systems that maintain the elder's current functioning.
(6) Triangulation/ scapegoating: Utilization of a person to avoid other family issues, usually highly emotional ones.	Increased propensity to focus on an elder in family.	(a) Refocus attacks by redefining issues from elder to family. (b) Help family members to share responsibilities. (c) Introduction of others, e.g. home health aides. (d) Impose restraints to prevent abuse.
(7) Double binds: Trapping of individuals in family through distortions of communications.	Powerful message can have severe effect on elder.	(a) Clarifying messages sent and received. (b) Reframing negative responses and resistance to positive actions. (c) Separating individuals in the family.

Figure 8.1. Key Concepts and Interventions Relative to the Older Family
SOURCE: Tonti, M., & Silverstone, B. (1985). Services to Families of the Elderly. In Monk, A. (Ed.). *Handbook of Gerontological Services*. New York: Van Nostrand Reinhold. Reprinted by permission.

or her interpretation of the reason behind a particular complaint. *Offering alternative solutions* to dealing with a problem or complaint can be attempted if the practitioner believes the older person is receptive to such suggestions and can accept the fact that his or her previous efforts at problem resolution have not worked. Finally, and as a last resort, confrontation may be turned to. *Confrontation* entails pointing out inconsistencies in the older person's behavior without being unduly critical. The latter technique should be considered in only those cases where older clients are not particularly defensive. It should not be practiced simply because practitioners are impatient or frustrated with a lack of movement on the part of a client.

Reframing problems or complaints for clients often represents a major activity of the practitioner engaged in counseling. Reframing entails expanding the focus of the problem so as to allow for solutions that might otherwise have not been considered (Bumagin and Hirn, 1990). For example, in home care, real hostility about how the home health aide cooks or makes the bed may really be anger about lost control and independence. Reframing the problem can help the older person understand this.

Preparing older persons for the time when services may come to an end can be a pivotal aspect of the counseling process. Sensitive termination planning is especially critical for vulnerable clients experiencing a difficult time with loss and dependence. It is not unusual for problems to arise in the service plan near the point of termination as clients express their fear and reluctance to deal with yet another loss, that of the departure of staff of the home care agency (see Chapter 9). Good counseling around termination entails the ability to remove yourself from the situation without causing emotional injury to the older person. This is more likely to happen when termination is dealt with early on in the relationship between client and agency. It is also addressed by setting a finite time frame for service (which is, of course, subject to periodic modification), ensuring that the critical connection is forged between client and agency rather than client and practitioner, and building up alternative informal and formal supports prior to your departure.

To summarize the discussion of home care counseling techniques and methods the following practice guidelines are offered:

1. *Whenever possible make goal agreements with the older person.* The goals that are set should be limited and very realistic. The intent behind conservative goal setting is the rapid establishment of a new point of equilibrium between person and environment.

2. *Deal with anxiety by means of preventive planning.* Impending losses should be anticipated as much as possible and supports provided in their place.

3. *Deal with periods of panic by promoting ventilation of fear and anger, providing reassurance, and balancing the offering of emotional and concrete supports.* Major changes in personality are not likely during these periods and should not be sought.

4. *Focus on accomplishments and other positive attainments in the life of the person.* This process of "selective reminiscence" aims to strengthen ego integrity and promotes a refocusing on aspects of the older person's life of which he or she may not be aware.

9

Case Closing/Termination

This chapter considers the final phases of geriatric case practice in home health care. Attention is given to the circumstances under which case termination is likely to occur as well as the methods and techniques that the case practitioner has available to conduct the closing of a home care case. In addition, guidelines for engaging in responsible case follow-up and follow-through are discussed.

Home health care cases do not remain open indefinitely. In fact, a multitude of factors are present in the service arena that dictate that a case practitioner's client load will fluctuate considerably even over short periods of time. It is therefore essential that home health care workers be prepared for the inevitability of frequent and often unexpected case terminations and, in turn, be skilled in the methods by which effective case closing is achieved.

Case termination is brought on by a variety of circumstances. Most tend to be related to worsening client status either in the physical, psychological, functional, or economic domains of an older person's life. Termination, however, may also be brought on by influences in the environment that are not directly related to the condition of the older person. Circumstances under which termination occurs may therefore be categorized as: (a) those where service termination is due to alteration in client status—for example, client-centered factors; and (b) those where service termination is the result of situationally or environmentally induced factors and are thus not in response to client change or need per se.

Circumstances Related to Changes in Client Status

Termination may be brought on by improvement in the client's condition such that he or she no longer requires assistance. Similarly, the client may eventually be in need of a lower level of care because of gradual improvement from an acute illness or accident (i.e., the older person may no longer need the services of a professional social worker, nurse, or home health aide but, rather, could be satisfied with receiving the support of a friendly visitor or intermittent chore and escort service). Less intensive services may be unavailable from a particular home health care agency or more appropriately delivered by another agency.

Although not the most common of the client-centered factors, improvement in the older person's condition is often overlooked, much to the detriment of the client's well-being. As members of a society unduly focused on the deterioration that accompanies the aging process, home care professionals may neglect to recognize an increased capacity for autonomous functioning on the part of the client. The harm caused by such an oversight extends beyond unnecessary dependence to encompass possible premature or avoidable physical deterioration, resignation, and depression as in the following case:

> After being discharged from the hospital where he received treatment for the effects of a stroke, Mr. Howard returned to his home. The services of a home health agency were engaged because of his inability to carry out many routine activities without assistance. In keeping with the case plan, Mr. Howard's aide bathed and dressed him daily. As he recovered, he began to attempt simple personal hygiene routines and to put on some articles of clothing. Obviously unable to do these chores perfectly or quickly initially, the aide would interrupt his efforts and complete the activities herself, frustrating the client. No case plan modifications were made. After having his attempts thwarted again and again, Mr. Howard became resigned to a life of dependence for personal needs, although unnecessary. Recognizing that significant recovery from his stroke would not become a reality, he gradually slipped into a depression. Neither the home health aide nor the supervisor

were initially able to determine why Mr. Howard's condition was seemingly deteriorating. It was only after a careful reassessment of Mr. Howard's behavior and the factors leading to the depression that the case practitioner was able to recognize what had transpired. An altered care plan was immediately put into effect and shortly thereafter Mr. Howard's depression lifted.

Termination of service may be indicated because greater client care becomes necessary. More intensified service needs, such as institutional long-term care, hospice care, or hospital treatment may arise when clients are experiencing deterioration due to an accident or chronic illness decline. Under these circumstances the home health care agency will not be equipped to provide the altered set of intensified services. Termination under these circumstances may also occur if the home care program does not have the new set of home health care interventions required by the client. For instance, the older person who is no longer able to self-medicate (e.g., administer his or her own insulin injections) may require home health care personnel who are authorized to engage in medication administration. Under these circumstances the agency that employs home attendants and social workers but not nurses and nurses aides may have to close the case because its staff is only authorized to supervise medication regimens.

In effect, decrements in client status may bring about termination of services, not because home health care becomes an inappropriate service strategy but, rather, because a particular agency's service repertoire is unable to respond to a client's altered set of home care needs.

Cases may close not because of change in intensity of needed care, which, in fact, may remain stable, but, rather, because change occurs in the status of a client's informal support network. That is, formal home health care services may no longer be needed because family members, friends, and/or neighbors have stepped forward to offer help. For example, a client may move in with a daughter or son, or a client's niece may establish regularized contact with the older person and begin to perform those functions that the case practitioner or aide had been formerly performing. While it is more likely that a blood relative would take on the responsibility of care, it could also be a close friend or a younger person who agrees to engage in a home sharing arrangement and provide supportive services in exchange for room and board.

It is not infrequent that home health cases close due to the death of a client. The demise of an older person receiving service may be predictable or totally unexpected given the complexities of illness in old age.

While the ability to provide short-term supportive service to bereaved family members varies from one agency to another, it should be considered a part of the basic service package whenever feasible. Following the death of a loved one, families may find it difficult to negotiate the complex system that must be faced in order to make necessary arrangements. Home health staff can provide a valuable function by providing guidance with both tasks (e.g., arranging for termination of benefits) and emotional issues (e.g., allowing for ventilation of feelings). In the event that the agency is unable to provide such services, it is imperative that an appropriate referral be made when deemed necessary.

Finally, a home health care case may terminate due simply to client dissatisfaction. The older person in this case can express displeasure with the quality of services being provided, the competency of home health personnel, or the configuration of the service package that has been made available.

Circumstances Related to Environmentally Induced Factors

The classic example of this type of case closing is when service is discontinued due to an agency's regulatory requirements. If service is being covered via third-party payments (e.g., Medicare or Medicaid), termination may be brought about when the client no longer meets medical and/or financial requirements for coverage and could be satisfied by receiving medical social services, homemaker assistance, custodial or maintenance care, or assistance in performing the activities of daily living (i.e., shopping, cleaning, cooking, dressing, etc.). Similarly, services may be discontinued if the agency providing home care is funded through the Older Americans Act because care is necessarily time limited and the coverage period has come to an end, or the client may come to require more hours of coverage than can be authorized.

Service may come to a close because the elderly client or the family feels that the amount that can be expended for home care has been reached. In this situation the client may choose to avoid depleting all of his or her assets in order to become eligible for Medicaid-subsidized home health care services (i.e., spending down to Medicaid eligibility levels). This type of termination is more likely to occur when the elder is purchasing home health care at market value through a proprietary (for-profit) system of service.

In the age of the time-limited project, service has been known to terminate simply because the agency providing care is forced to close its doors. Defunding of a demonstration and research project causes the closing of cases in which need for care may well still persist, but because the designated funding period has passed, supports are withdrawn. This category of case termination can be especially difficult to deal with because the demonstration service is frequently one that is unavailable elsewhere. The dilemma of providing critically needed care to a vulnerable, at-risk elderly population, knowing it will be withdrawn at a specified future date, is considered in detail by Weinstein and Zlotnick (1986) in their review of the termination of the New York City's Department for the Aging's Home Care Project. The Home Care Project was one of several federally supported research and demonstration projects operated during the early and mid-1980s throughout the United States. The importance of preparing early on for case discharge in the case of the time-limited program cannot be emphasized enough. The issues to be concerned about are addressed later in this chapter when case closing technique, follow-up, and follow-through are discussed.

Clients may be required to stop receiving service because their financial status has changed to one that does not fall within the boundaries of eligibility of a particular home health care program. For example, the person may stop being a private pay client and become eligible for Medicaid or Medicare home care, but the agency to which they are attached is not third-party reimbursable or not a certified provider of Medicare or Medicaid home health care services.

There is the rare case where the elderly client's financial status improves because a new source of financial support becomes available (e.g., a pension or annuity plan becomes effective). They may then be required to discontinue a subsidized service and move to being a private purchaser of care.

Agencies have been known to become dissatisfied with a client and ultimately bring service to a premature close. Program participants may be excessively difficult, demanding, or abusive; they or their families and friends may repeatedly sabotage the case plan, or a client-worker match may be impossible to engineer successfully (see, for example, Kaye, 1985a; Browdie & Turwoski, 1986). Elder clients who suffer from extremely disruptive bouts of paranoia and related psychological disturbances can accelerate decisions to close a case on the part of the home health agency.

> Miss Silverman had been receiving services from a particular home health care agency for more than a year without complication. Gradually, she began evidencing unusual behaviors such as questioning the location of an article of clothing she had just put in the closet, frequently claiming to have lost money, and showing concern about the suspicious-looking people entering her apartment building. Although not a problem to the aide, she appropriately made note of the situation to her supervisor and was told to continue to monitor the client's behavior and report any changes. With time, this behavior escalated to a point where Miss Silverman was falsely accusing the aide, among others, of stealing her clothing, money, and other possessions as well as of being in collusion with the suspicious sorts in the building. The supervisor, recognizing the client's paranoid ideation, arranged for a full medical and psychological evaluation at the local clinic where Miss Silverman was seen regularly to determine the origin of the inappropriate behavior. The results indicated no physical impairment, but, rather, a disturbance of a psychiatric nature. Attempts to treat the condition with medication proved fruitless. The behavior became so extreme that the agency could no longer subject its staff to working under such conditions. Termination became necessary, and an appropriate referral was made without disruption of service, benefiting both the client and the home health agency.

Finally, the severing of a client-worker bond that cannot be repaired may force the closing of a case. A home health care worker who is especially loved by an elderly client may leave the agency. Subsequent replacements inevitably fail for a variety of reasons, usually because the new worker lacks some quality that the original staff person displayed. Such case plans that require constant change can prove to be seriously disruptive for the small-scale agency in particular. In these instances case termination is often the only possible alternative.

The various circumstances outlined above that can lead to case termination suggest that a series of interventive issues and strategies will have to be considered during the termination phase. In particular it is important to make appropriate referral and transfer plans well in advance to allow for continuity of care with the least disruption. Under certain circumstances there is inadequate time for such preparation. Should such a situation arise, staff are forced to manage referral and transfer in a brief period of time, but it is imperative that quality client care remain the primary goal. Of course the issues that the case practitioner must be prepared to deal with and the arsenal of skills that he or she will be able to draw upon will vary depending on the specific circumstances leading to termination.

The extent to which termination counseling takes place also depends in part on the particular training that the case practitioner has undergone as well as the nature of the agency performance description by which he or she is compelled to abide. The willingness of the elderly client to engage in termination planning combined with the skills of the case practitioner and the willingness of the home health agency to allow the worker to engage in this kind of professional assistance combine to determine the intensity and quality of care provided during this phase of service.

Termination Issues

Any and all of the following case closing issues may arise during termination.

1. *Feelings of Personal Loss.* The withdrawal of a home health care worker may represent the loss of a family member or close intimate friend for the older person. In many cases home care personnel come to fulfill quasi-family like functions in the eyes of the older client. This is especially the case for the isolated and vulnerable older person. The severing of these powerful affective ties can result in the client entering a period of "bereavement" in which actual psychological mourning takes place. This eventuality needs to be anticipated and worked through by the case practitioner, especially when the client-worker relationship is known to be a close and intimate one.

By the same token, broken attachments between worker and client may evoke emotional stress reactions on the part of the home care service provider who, in turn, may require opportunities for ventilating feelings pertaining to service termination. The breaking of personal bonds can be difficult for everyone concerned. Feelings of pain, abandonment, and anxiety over separation are not rare in such cases (National HomeCaring Council, 1982). The death of a client can also be expected to illicit a mourning response in the home health care worker who has been providing service over an extended period of time. (See Silverstone & Burack-Weiss, 1983a, for a review of the practice difficulties posed by transfer and termination when working with the frail elderly.)

2. *Anxiety Over Instrumental Loss.* The client may be justifiably worried over the impending loss of one or more home health care services that comprised his or her care package. The loss of concrete services, of formal service supports, requires explanation in clear terms as to which supportive care interventions will no longer be available to the individual and which, if any, will replace those withdrawn.

3. *Transitional Stress.* Similar to relocation trauma for the older person facing institutionalization, it is not unusual for transitional stress to accompany a change in life-style for the home care client. Home care transitional stress rises out of the older person's fear of the unknown (i.e., life without the home health care worker who had been coming to the client's house two or three times a week) as well as fear of impending isolation and loss of emotional support. Loss of service represents for some simply another landmark or life marker confirming their own aging, mortality, and impending demise from which there is no return. Case practitioners must not downplay the potential significance of transitional stress just as the implications of relocation trauma should not be underestimated for the older person facing institutionalization. Each can be severely disabling or even fatal under certain circumstances. Adequate advance notice of termination plans and systematic attention to easing transitional stress is essential.

4. *Functional, Physical, and Mental Decline.* Case practitioners need to be prepared to deal with the eventuality of deteriorating client

health status at the point of termination. Health counseling that centers on understanding the changes taking place in the individual's physical and mental state and its impact on functional capacity is necessary. Reality testing needs to be encouraged at the same time that a reasonable dose of hope is injected into the client's frame of thinking about the future. The practitioner should also be prepared to discuss the relationship between worsened client health and the ability of the service network to serve them adequately. The eventual need to be institutionalized may have to be raised, as well as the importance of preparing the client for this eventuality in order to make the process a less painful and abrupt one.

5. *Dependency and Aging.* Maintaining dignity and self-esteem in the face of functional decline is very difficult. Maintaining such dignity during what may be an undesired withdrawal of service is an even greater test of character and personal strength. Client achievement of these ends should be among the practice goals of the case practitioner during this phase of service delivery. If, on the other hand, client change is for the better, as in the case of Mr. Howard, assistance may well be needed in helping the individual to regain confidence in his or her capacity for a higher level of self-sufficiency and autonomous behavior.

In the case of a change in the older person's financial status, attention may need to be directed toward issues of Medicaid as welfare and charity. For many, especially the elderly, subsidized care carries with it a powerful stigma, including a sense of undesired dependence on the government and compliance in the face of public home health care agency intervention. The idea of being means-tested may be degrading in the eyes of a client who had been paying a fee-for-service up to that point. The need to "spend-down" to Medicaid eligibility levels may be initially unacceptable to many individuals. The erosion of one's financial cushion in life, one's life savings, frequently gives rise to a lost sense of freedom, feelings of anger, resentment, and powerlessness. The home health care worker has the responsibility of anticipating such feelings in his or her clients and intervening in ways that help the person feel more in control of his or her own life and the decisions that impact on the client's situations (Silverstone & Burack-Weiss, 1983a).

6. *Service Awareness and Utilization.* For those elderly clients who will require alternative service supports subsequent to the withdrawal of care, case practitioners have the responsibility of assessing levels of service awareness, knowledge, and utilization. Clients need to be assisted in understanding alternate interventive strategies and their accompanying eligibility criteria as well as being offered helpful information concerning how to negotiate and access the alternative service. Clients should also be assisted in understanding the intent of the alternative service or services, including the rationale behind moving to more or less intensive interventions based on an individual's functional status. Such counseling may entail a discussion of the abilities and limitations of various personnel in the home health care service network as well as the skills of accessing the service network and the appropriateness of one entitlement or benefit over another.

The genuine limitations of home health care need also to be considered. That is, clients should be helped to understand that home health care may come to be an inappropriate form of aid at some point in their lives.

7. *Family Relations.* The relationship between the older person and his or her family (or other social supports) can surface as an issue requiring attention during case termination. This will more likely be the case in those instances where family members are having their older relative move in with them or where a relative has agreed to fulfill one or more home care functions formerly performed by the service provider. Issues for consideration include: a) the need for privacy, b) respect for others, c) role alterations and the potential for role reversal, d) territoriality, e) potential for infantilization, and f) the possibility of promoting excessive dependency. Dysfunctional, unhealthy caretaker-elder relationships can frequently emerge when the provision of home care type services are being performed for the first time by one's relatives. Case closing may demand both individual and family counseling in order to ensure that expectations, roles, and behaviors are clarified, understood, and maintained over time by all concerned.

The problems associated with territoriality and respect for the life-style of the elderly client and the individual or individuals providing care are frequently central matters requiring attention. A willingness to compromise is essential for all parties involved.

8. *Death and Bereavement*. In those instances where termination is brought about by the death of a client, bereavement counseling may be in order for the surviving family members. Realistically speaking, this should be a short-term service if provided by the home health care case practitioner. Frequently, referral to a family service agency or independent therapist is in order as such assistance is not a common service provided by a home health care program. Case practitioners, therefore, need to have some knowledge of family counseling agencies in the community in order that an appropriate referral can be made. (*Hospice Care*, a volume in the **Geriatric Case Practice Training Series** exploring case practice in hospices, considers the elements of bereavement counseling in detail.)

9. *Dysfunctional Behavior*. The case practitioner has some responsibility to confront the disruptive client, even at the point of case closing. This assumes the ability by the professional to recognize and identify potential dysfunctional behavior in the older person (e.g., mental illness, depression, paranoia, delusional states, psychoses, etc.), as in the case of Miss Silverman as well as those factors that may contribute to or exacerbate the disruptive state such as improper use of medications, malnutrition, environmental or social stress, and so on. The importance of being able to identify those mental health services that the clients might avail themselves of and to offer such recommendations in a nonthreatening manner to clients can be a real test of the skills of the home health care case practitioner.

In addition, the case practitioners have the responsibility of being mindful of recognizing when the point has been reached where the elderly client is a hazard to himself, herself, or others. At such times significant others should be notified and a modified plan of care devised that entails a more intensified set of service supports (e.g., adult protective services, institutional care or the like).

Case Closing—Follow-Up to Follow-Through

In actuality most home health care agencies do not have the staff time nor mandate to provide extensive follow-up services subsequent to case termination. Agencies that accept governmental, third-party payments have caseloads that preclude follow-up beyond the minimum required standards. Proprietary agencies, on the other hand, may not view post-termination follow-up as being in the organization's best interests in the absence of additional fees being levied.

Regardless of the agency's auspice, responsible postservice delivery at the minimum encompasses a series of basic follow-up actions. Case practitioners in the home health care field have the professional responsibility of ensuring their timely and effective implementation. It is likely that these actions will be more successfully performed if they are begun early on. This requires that termination be anticipated well in advance and the required actions carried out in systematic fashion. Early termination planning provides the practitioner with an opportunity to address potential client resistance to the termination of service or difficulties associated with transition to a new service package. Inadequate attention to this phase of the service sequence encourages the likelihood of poor client adjustment and unnecessary stress and strain resulting from the withdrawal of service (see, for example, Kaye, 1985a).

Minimum Standards for Case Termination

The following action steps represent minimum standards of professional practitioner behavior in the face of service termination:

1. To provide the elderly client with referral information required to secure an alternate set of needed supportive care services;
2. To notify the client's significant social supports of the case closing, anticipated client needs, and recommended referral services;
3. To cooperate with the agency to which the client has been referred by providing any needed case information (assuming that approval for release of said information has been granted by the former client);
4. To assure the client that access to the home health care agency may be achieved at a later date if circumstances require and permit it; and
5. To maintain an up-to-date set of client records and essential information on closed cases, including all referral data in the event that there is future contact with the individual or another service provider.

Where agency resources allow it, case practitioners may engage in more active and intensified referral and follow-through functions, including a set of actions that approximate those of the case manager or case coordinator. These include:

1. Making the actual client referral and ensuring that the referral is successfully acted upon by all parties concerned, that is, guaranteeing that the referral agreement is arrived at and implemented;

2. Providing at least one follow-up contact with the former client and/or his or her significant others in order to ensure the smooth transition of the elderly client from one service status to the next. The case practitioner engages in short-term monitoring focusing on the adjustment of the individual to the new service package. Follow-up contact can include as well the performance of a nurturing function for the older person's informal supports, providing him or her with clues as to the anticipated future needs of the client and describing strategies whereby the informal supports can be of assistance to the older person;

3. Conducting a follow-up assessment of client status at a specified time interval, including an evaluation of the older person's health and social status and the adequacy of the new service through contact with the agency to which the client was referred; and

4. In the event of the death of the client, carrying out follow-up contact with the surviving relatives and any other social supports of the person. Assistance in this situation might entail providing appropriate referrals to any needed services (e.g., support groups and self-help organizations, legal assistance organizations that deal with estates and wills, and counseling services that specialize in bereavement difficulties).

Appendix A:
Model Fieldwork Assignments

The following are model fieldwork assignments designed to help new practitioners develop the skills and knowledge necessary for doing geriatric case practice in home health care. Much of the content of the volume is reflected in the objectives of the assignments. The assignments identify learning tasks, offer example activities that provide opportunities to master the tasks and knowledge, and suggest criteria that could be used to evaluate the level of mastery achieved. As organized, the model assignments can be used in structured or self-directed instruction. The model fieldwork assignments contained in this appendix were developed as part of a larger training project called Mastery-Based Curriculum Utilization for Geriatric Case Practice.

The Geriatric Case Practice Model:
Some Background on Its Development

The Administration of Aging awarded the George Warren Brown School of Social Work, Washington University (St. Louis, MO), a grant to develop a training program in geriatric case practice titled Mastery-Based Curriculum Utilization for Geriatric Case Practice. The grant supported the development of a portable curriculum constructed so that it could easily be incorporated into existing training programs, yet complete enough to stand on its own.

The term *Geriatric Case Practice* has been coined to distinguish this form of geriatric practice from other approaches, a moniker that not only distinguishes the domain of practice, but also highlights a distinctive training approach.

At the heart of the training is competency-based learning. This approach recognizes that many generic courses and field opportunities can be used to develop specific practice skills related to work with the elderly across the continuum provided that the proper learning tasks are identified and supplemental materials are made available. Such learning modules could then be used by instructors and students to offer specialized training opportunities within the context of more generic courses and fieldwork settings.

The curriculum development effort included the organization of classroom materials and fieldwork opportunities for the different service settings forming the continuum of care. Classroom elements included readings, audiovisual materials, and exercises.

To help structure the field placements and ensure quality field instruction, model fieldwork assignments for five settings were developed. These five settings correspond to the five volumes in the **Geriatric Case Practice Training Series** that focus on field settings:

1. Case management in geriatric community-based settings
2. Work in acute care hospitals and geriatric assessment units
3. Practice in home-health care settings
4. Case practice in nursing homes
5. Work in hospice programs

The volumes in the series focus on working with distinct groups of elderly and their families across the range of service settings comprising the continuum of care: (a) the independent elderly living in the community, (b) the ill elderly in acute care medical settings and the role of multidisciplinary geriatric assessment, (c) home-delivered and community-based services directed toward the frail elderly continuing to reside in the community but requiring home care, (d) nursing home residents and their care, and (e) the dying elderly and their need for hospice care.

As part of the project, knowledgeable practitioners were called upon to form working task groups to identify the skills and items of knowledge needed to effectively operate in these different types of service arenas. The materials drafted by these practitioners form the foundation from which the following model assignments are based.

Use of the Model Fieldwork Assignments

The use of field training permits the development of skills in a natural setting. Learning through performance has always been a vital aspect of training. It demands active involvement and besides teaching specific technical skills, forces the application and integration of knowledge into practice.

The sequence of field placements within the training model mirrored the continuum of care available in the service system. The sequence itself structures the learning opportunities by typically exposing students to populations of elderly clients varying greatly in levels of independence, physical mobility, and health. While constructed within the training program to serve as a sequenced series of placements, any of the model field assignments can be used alone.

The model home health care assignments echo the skills and information specified in the volume. They have been developed to guide the learning experience, help clarify the intended learning objectives, and specify how competencies may be evaluated by field supervisors or by practitioners themselves. The model assignments for home health care reflect the natural abilities and opportunities provided by the setting.

Within the context of the model fieldwork assignments, the targeted skills and knowledge are termed learning objectives and organized under three broad groupings: (a) Professional Knowledge, (b) Administrative Knowledge and Skills, and (c) Program Objectives.

Professional Knowledge

Learning Objective

1. To gain knowledge and understanding about:
    a. Disease symptoms
    b. Medication
    c. Prognosis
    d. Medicare
    e. Medicaid
    f. Third-party pay insurance
    g. Personal care
    h. Chore housekeeper
    i. General home health care guidelines and program regulations
    j. Durable medical equipment—types and usage
    k. Mental health—services, problems

    l. Impact of illness on patient and family
    m. Dysfunctioning family relationships with patients
    n. Use of data and research in the development of services

Learning Experiences

1. Review literature as it applies to the home health care setting and construct annotated bibliography
2. Participate in staff conferences; in-service training. (Consider the use of videotapes used by agency for training of nurses, other professionals.)
3. Attend seminars and workshops and review videotapes on subjects listed
4. Review guidelines, regulations—federal, state, and individual insurance contracts—that affect services provided by the assigned agency
5. Be assigned a caseload representative of the problems listed

Criteria for Evaluation

1. Complete an in-service presentation or present your supervisor with written documentation on assigned cases. Supervisor evaluation will be based on the following:
    a. Information about equipment, referral process, and if availability of services is accurate and complete
    b. Define source regulation or insurance plan source to verify statements regarding financial eligibility
    c. Produce evidence of research—bibliography, articles reviewed, books, flyers, bulletins, brochures—that were used as a basis for information in developing presentations, announcements, brochures, and uses the references appropriately
2. Documentation in record reflects guidelines of regulations, bulletins re: home health service. Record includes:
    a. Reason for referral
    b. Treatment information
    c. Goals of session
    d. Plan for future visits

Learning Objective

2. Further developing and enhancing the ability to be self-reliant and flexible; adaptable in the home health setting
    a. Using assertiveness as a professional in this setting

    b. Assuming responsibility for decisions in planning for services with the client

    c. Understanding and using the role of advocacy

Learning Experiences

1. Supervisor requires case practitioner to process record, audiotape or videotape at least one experience that demonstrates the decision-making ability of the practitioner re: service delivery involving the client.
2. Review record documentation, prioritize information in order to make decisions before seeing the client. This process is reviewed with supervisor for comments and suggestions.
3. Review the services rendered to the client from beginning to close. It is suggested that audiotapes, videotapes, or process recording be produced at:
   a. Opening
   b. Halfway through the case
   c. Close of case if time allows for this. In any event, the initial assessment can be examined with practitioner-supervisor review regarding decision-making
4. Caseload should represent samples of issues listed in this objective.
5. Practitioner and supervisor will examine changes in the system. (Crisis management if this occurs during practicum.)

Criteria for Evaluation

1. Process recordings or audiotapes document practitioner's ability to:
   a. Initiate responses
   b. Summarize and comment on material client gives in a direct way without offending client
   c. Identify service plan with client, asking for input and comments
   d. Reinforce positive responses and build on strengths
   e. Offer client alternatives, respecting his right to refuse any or all services
   f. Motivate client to carry out plan of care
   g. Terminate interview/relationship with ease
   h. Suggest follow-up care to appropriate resources
2. In management of a crisis the practitioner is able to:
   a. Observe/assess situation accurately
   b. Carry on responsibilities despite changes that take place
   c. Prioritize time, direct efforts relative to client needs, agency assignments

    d. Consider role of support to others when a crisis occurs
3. Practitioner is able to identify and adjust to changes in the care plan, responding to input, and decisions of others regarding new problems that become known during the treatment period.

Learning Objective

3. Ability to develop/maintain professional support systems in home health

Learning Experiences

1. Review those relevant organizations that meet regularly for the purpose of networking in home health
2. Review with supervisor what agency meetings are of special value in home health for purposes of further developing expertise in this field.;
3. Review decision-making process to determine how requests re- garding career development issues are accomplished and what money and time are allocated for this purpose
4. Identify what is considered personal career development for which personal resources can be used
5. Establish an information file, with addresses and telephone numbers of those professionals, who have been helpful in assisting practitioner during job. It is recommended that a copy of this information be made available to the agency—this type of file with important agency numbers would also be helpful if the agency does not already have such a file.

Criteria for Evaluation

1. Report on role of agency, costs agency is willing to incur for professional training of staff, organization—showing evidence of source of decision (budget item, administrative decision, etc.).
2. Implement the plan of care using identified network of professionals. Client records should contain documentation of contacts: who, what, where, when.
3. Completeness of this information that identifies key individuals who can be called on for direct assistance in implementing a plan of care
4. Complete an evaluation of relevant conferences attended while in training, making recommendations re: speakers, content, and learning objectives and whether agency benefited and should offer future support

Administrative Knowledge and Skills

Learning Objective

A-1. To gain knowledge/understanding of the agency's overall organizational structure (formal/informal)

Learning Experiences

1. Review literature that addresses administration, management, and organizational structure in home health agencies
2. Review manuals and other organizational information that reflects administrative structure of the agency
3. Interview administrative personnel as to roles and responsibilities of individuals in management positions
4. As part of orientation training, interview/observe the administrator, examining daily responsibilities, duties, decision-making issues that are part of the job

Criteria for Evaluation

1. Follow chain of command when situation requires a decision
2. Identify who is in charge for what areas and whom to consult with in the absence of supervisor
3. Develop an informal flow chart; can determine allies in system who support professional decisions

Learning Objective

A-2. To gain knowledge/understanding of the agency's overall fiscal/budgetary process

Learning Experiences

1. Interview fiscal manager
2. Trace the flow of monies for reimbursement—one case each
    a. Medicare
    b. Medicaid
    c. Third-party pay

Criteria for Evaluation

1. Outline two cases and identify source of reimbursement. If there are no monies at all, what is the implication on care plan? Supervisor will evaluate:
   a. How the information was obtained
   b. If it was accurate
   c. If the information was utilized in the plan of care
   d. If the funding agency actually covered costs
2. Report on contacts, guidelines, criteria, general issues related to rate of reimbursement coverage
3. Knowledge about what questions to ask client and others to get necessary information to make decision

Learning Objective

A-3. To gain knowledge/understanding of the agency's mission

Learning Experiences

1. Review agency material, philosophy, minutes of board meetings for consistency, matching against actual practice
2. Review literature identifying four types of home health care agencies:
   a. Characteristics of each
   b. Regulations
   c. Differences in reporting and recording
3. If agency has a "special project," allow practitioner to be involved in planning and implementing project to observe how programming occurs in the organization.

Criteria for Evaluation

1. Outline in presentation covering the following information:
   a. Mission of agency
   b. Type of agency—what this means in program, funding, and reporting
   c. Population served
   d. History of the organization
2. Write a summary of information on assigned project outlining:
   a. Reason for assignment
   b. Methodology utilized
   c. Source and summary of information gathered
   d. Plan for implementation

e. Recommendations

Report is sent through appropriate channels as outlined in agency structure. Evaluation is made on the completeness of the summary report.

3. Document gaps in lines of authority where breakdown seemed to occur to supervisor

Learning Objective

A-4. To further develop abilities and to demonstrate skills in training agency personnel—professionals and paraprofessionals

Learning Experiences

1. Design/conduct an in-service meeting on one of the following:
   a. Community resources
   b. New services
   c. Aging process
   d. Communication skills
   e. Other—please list
2. Develop/conduct a support group for paraprofessionals
3. Research regulations/requirements of agency contracts
4. Conduct a program for agency personnel on these issues

Criteria for Evaluation

1. Presentation is evaluated on:
   a. Organization of material presented
   b. Ability to present material in a clear, concise manner, in language understood by audience
   c. Questions by audience—Did questions indicate audience generally understood issues?
   d. Number of participants attending session
   e. Information provided on evaluation form: Did the participant learn anything? Were there comments on the presenter's style and ability to communicate ideas?

Learning Objective

A-5. To gain knowledge about the role of the social worker as a consultant to systems and home health staff in areas of:
   a. Noncompliance regarding treatment plan

b. Family relationships
c. Community services—availability of services

Learning Experiences

1. Participate in case conferences—assist coordinator in writing the outcomes of one conference following agency procedures
2. Consider audiotaping and/or role playing the role of consultant in home health care social work
3. Examine what role the social worker has in relation to specific cases assigned. (If possible, report to group on issues listed in objective and how they affect treatment plans.)

Criteria for Evaluation

1. Could the trainee identify the role the social worker played in changing the direction of the team on one case reviewed? What specific changes were approved and why this happened?

Learning Objective

A-6. To develop the ability to act in the consultant role in the home health care agency

Learning Experiences

1. Participate in the management of homemakers, personal care workers, other paraprofessionals, and volunteers utilized by the agency in service delivery
2. Evaluate the role and effectiveness of service delivery
3. Participate in special projects established by the agency

Criteria for Evaluation

1. Supervisor, observing practitioner, evaluates:
    a. Ability to communicate with others—getting the message over
    b. Plan of care has been adjusted, reflecting ideas about service delivery in the case
    c. Ability to explain to nurses and other personnel why service plans are not always implemented as scheduled
    d. Ability to be creative in getting cooperation of community resources and agency personnel

Learning Objective

A-7. To gain knowledge about the basic principles of marketing/public relations as it relates to:
   a. Overall view of agency operations
   b. Planning in a home health agency
   c. Developing the marketplace—targeting service areas
   d. Analysis of statistics in planning services

Learning Experiences

1. Participate in in-service training of marketing personnel
2. Interview hospital personnel about marketing techniques
3. Observe other field representatives who market products
4. Spend one day observing individual(s) responsible for public relations and/or marketing
5. Review overall marketing plan of agency, if one is available
6. Choose a local community resource, such as a senior center, and explain the services of assigned agency to participants
7. Develop a tool for evaluating agency marketing techniques. Review and analyze tools used elsewhere for this purpose
8. Participate in intake, checking incoming calls—Where did the client learn about the service? Other relevant information that will help evaluate marketing direction

Criteria for Evaluation

1. When practitioner makes a presentation, supervisor evaluates:
   a. Content of material presented. Was it relevant, accurate, covered issues related to agency services?
   b. Style—Was he or she comfortable, appropriately dressed? Could he or she answer questions posed?
   c. Creativity in presentation
   d. Planning for presentation—Was homework done?
   e. Was the presentation information reinforced with written information summarizing presentation issues?
   f. Examine audience evaluation form completed by participants?

Learning Objective

A-8. To gain knowledge about supervision of professionals, paraprofessional staff who are part of home health care services

Learning Experiences

1. Review literature about supervision:
    a. Responsibilities process
    b. Roles
    c. Expectations
    d. Authority—in health settings and in home health settings
2. Interview/observe the role of the supervisor
3. Sit in on an evaluation process
4. Assist agency personnel responsible for supervision of these workers in supervisory activities

Criteria for Evaluation

1. Write a report that:
    a. Defines the role of supervision in program reviewed
    b. Demonstrates who does supervision
    c. Illustrates how supervisory contacts are documented
    d. Tells what information is reviewed with supervisee
    e. Refers to state/agency guidelines for supervisory visits

Learning Objective

A-9. To gain knowledge about the role of the social worker as part of the home health team

Learning Experiences

1. Review guidelines on role of social work as a professional service in relation to primary disciplines in this field
2. Interview other professional personnel, asking about their views of the role of the social worker
3. Examine case records to determine when social work is called in on a case and for what reason
4. Process a case conference to determine if and when social work has a leadership role—What kind of leadership do others see the social worker as important in implementing the plan of care? Do all agree?

Criteria for Evaluation

1. Explain to others:
    a. Criteria for referral to social worker
    b. What services can be provided

    c. How often can services be provided?
    d. Role of social work in home care
    e. When services are terminated and for what reason
    f. Channels of communication with social worker
    g. Goals of social work in home care

Program Objectives

Learning Objective

P-1. To gain knowledge about the assessment process as it is utilized in home health services

Learning Experiences

1. Review literature for assessment tools utilized in this field
2. Review agency guidelines, federal and state requirements relative to documentation of information gathered
3. Review with supervisor the purpose of an assessment when developing a treatment plan
4. Review agency records and social work recording to learn about style and essential information that is documented on agency forms
5. Develop a personalized individual outline that can be used when interviewing begins

Criteria for Evaluation

1. Demonstrate understanding of the following:
    a. General guidelines defining the role of the "qualified social worker" in home health care
    b. State guidelines, including bulletins, regarding social casework
2. Show evidence of having attended in-service orientation and of having reviewed manuals relating to assessment tool used by the agency
    d. Participated in the internal audit review process of agency charts —especially social work component

Learning Objective

P-2. To develop the ability to complete a comprehensive assessment identifying social work problems, interventions, goals

Learning Experiences

1. Introduced to assessment process in in-service training with supervisor
2. Review documentation in records, examining other assessments completed by other disciplines
3. Review assessments completed by social work to become acquainted with social work process
4. Observe supervisor completing assessment, keeping notes on interview process
5. Participate in the assessment process with the supervisor
6. Supervisor observes an assessment reviewing the process, and providing feedback on areas of strength and areas needing improvement

Criteria for Evaluation

1. Complete an independent assessment where the supervisor evaluates the following items:
   a. Is the reason for referral identified following guidelines listed?
   b. Are goals identified in the session with the client?
   c. Is the examination of client/caregiver/environment comprehensive?
   d. Does he or she have the ability to establish rapport?
   e. Is the client able to understand why social service is needed, who pays the bill, and what services are available in the community?
   f. When referrals are made, are they explained? Is client or family input and assistance explored?
   g. Is written documentation complete and accurate?

Learning Objective

P-3. To develop the ability to access and utilize community resources in order to implement treatment plans in home health

Learning Experiences

1. Review available on-site agency information on resources to become acquainted with files already established
2. Examine other data banks of I and R services (e.g., United Way, local AAA's, available directories, information gathered by student in previous placements)
3. Have assigned cases that require referral to community resources as part of the treatment plan to complete service goals

4. Complete a file of resources, updated for the agency, which can be utilized by others in the agency
5. Learn who the contact persons are who would be helpful in implement plan for client
6. Learn what questions are pertinent when trying to determine if the resource is available and helpful to client

Criteria for Evaluation

1. Ability to complete this implementation and follow-up on all assigned cases that require community resource referrals without ongoing supervision. Plan of care is reviewed and approved by the supervisor.
2. Documentation on implementation and follow-up is completed according to regulations and agency guidelines. All documentation is reviewed, approved, and signed off by agency supervisor.

Learning Objective

P-4. To gain knowledge about crisis intervention techniques when this is perceived as a recognized need in service delivery in home health

Learning Experiences

1. Become acquainted with type of crises clients may experience in home health care by interviewing members of other disciplines (especially nursing) and reading agency records that have identified this issue as part of service delivery
2. Review regulations and interpretations by intermediary responsible for reimbursement regarding crisis intervention as a recognized need
3. Review literature regarding techniques used for crisis intervention to determine what is relevant for use in this type of setting

Criteria for Evaluation

1. Write a definition of crisis intervention, identifying source of information, using a type of case in home health that requires crisis intervention techniques

Learning Objective

P-5. To develop the ability to utilize crisis intervention techniques when the case requires this type of intervention

Learning Experiences

1. When required in case assignments, be able to implement crisis intervention techniques and review with supervisor what techniques were used
2. Supervisor will review and comment on decisions, examining alternative strategies (if any were available)

Criteria for Evaluation

1. Demonstrate an understanding of what responsibilities are required of the worker when crisis intervention is required:
   a. Intake—establishing communication by telephone or direct service rapid assessment of the situation
   b. Case management service
   c. Closing of case
   d. Follow-up actions

Learning Objective

P-6. To gain knowledge about the use of short-term counseling techniques that may be utilized in this setting

Learning Experiences

1. Review literature about the terminology, definition, and use of short-term counseling techniques utilized as part of treatment planning in a home health setting
2. Review regulations regarding the use of counseling as defined in this setting, if reimbursement is expected under Medicare guidelines
3. Review with administrator and supervisor agency policy direction regarding this type of service—with or without reimbursement—private pay or other reimbursement mechanisms

Criteria for Evaluation

1. Ablity to define "short-term" counseling as it applies to home health including:
   a. Conditions appropriate for implementing service
   b. Most relevant problem to be examined
   c. Types of goals
   d. Projected number of visits
   e. Frequency of contacts

Learning Objective

P-7. To develop the ability to implement short-term counseling techniques when the case requires this type of intervention

Learning Experiences

1. Case assingments that may require this type of intervention—reviewing with supervisor the treatment plan, frequency, goals, expected outcomes

Criteria for Evaluation

1. Process record for at least one case. Supervisor will evaluate ability to:
   a. Elicit information about problem from client
   b. Specify most relevant problem
   c. Obtain client's cooperation and involvement
   d. Set goals that can be measured and completed

Learning Objective

P-8. To gain knowledge about guidelines established for documentation of social service information provided in service delivery

Learning Experiences

1. Review guidelines, documents, memos, agency policies, and procedures that relate to documenting information in the home health care record
2. The practitioner review and participate in the internal audit review process of records—should review at least three to five records following agency guidelines
3. All documentation should be reviewed and approved by agency supervisor throughout the practicum. Early reviews should include suggestions regarding:
   a. Prioritizing information
   b. Summarizing information
   c. Developing an integrated service plan that reflects reason for referral
   d. S/w intervention
   e. Goals or outcome
   f. Need for future visits

    g.   Input in case conferences

    h.   Team decisions that impact on social service delivery

4. If the agency has been denied reimbursement in the past for services provided, the practitioner should participate in the internal review process to understand reasons for denial regarding service plans, method of recording, or other such factors affecting agency operation

Criteria for Evaluation

1. Ability to record information, according to specified guidelines, in a clear and very concise manner, stating:
   a. Reason for referral
   b. Problems identified
   c. Goals of session strategies for implementing plan of care
   d. Projected numbers of future visits
   e. Recommendations for ongoing service

Supervisor approves and signs off on this documentation

Learning Objective

P-9. To improve communication skills with clients, families, other professionals, business groups in the community—emphasis is placed on telephone usage

Learning Experiences

1. Participate in the intake process to learn how to obtain relevant information, explain services to others, handle requests made of the agency that may or may not be able to be handled at the time
2. Request follow-up regarding services, evaluation of services, impact study to become comfortable with assessing a situation using this form of communication
3. Use the telephone in order to conduct assessments, keeping track of time, outcomes for agency, supervisory review
4. Participate in telecommunication training seminars available in the community through organizations such as Bell Telephone, AT&T, etc.

Criteria for Evaluation

1. Supervisor can observe practitioner while on the phone with a client, evaluating ability to:

    a.   Elicit Information

    b.   Assess client's ability to respond. For example, are there hearing problems? Can the client comprehend? Is there evidence of confusion?

    c.   Respond with courtesy

    d.   Establish basis for assessment

    e.   Obtain satisfactory closure

    f.   Establish goals for future contacts

Appendix B:
Home Health Care
Agency Service Forms

This appendix includes examples of various application, intake, referral, medication record, plan of care, agreement of treatment and release of information, and discharge summary forms used in home health care for the elderly. The have been reprinted with permission from Community Health Affiliates, Ardmore, PA, a private, not-for-profit home health care program.

PATTERN REFERRAL FORM

PATIENT REFERRAL FORM

Community Health
A F F I L I A T E S

Patient _____
           last   first

Address _____

_____ Zip Code _____

DOB _____ Phone _____

Sex: M F Lives Alone: Yes No Loc. _____

Marital Status: M W S Other

Race: Cau Black Other Spanish

Primary Caregiver _____

Address _____

_____ Phone _____

Primary Physician _____

Address _____

_____ Phone _____

Other Physician _____

Specialty _____ Phone _____

Hospital _____ from ____ to _____

Rehab _____ from ____ to _____

Other _____ from ____ to _____

Diet:

Activity:

Lab Work:

Ambulance:

Date of Referral _____ 1st Visit Date _____

Referred by _____

Agency _____ Phone _____

Taken by _____

Home Care# _____

Insurance: MC MA BC Other _____

Insur.# _____

2° Insur. _____

Fee: A____ B____ C____ D____ E____ F____

Patient#   codes

Dx _____ _____

_____ _____

_____ _____

Surgery _____ _____

_____ _____

Prognosis: Poor Fair Good Other _____

Course of Illness: (CC, V.S., PMH)

Services Ordered: Nursing_____ H.H.A_____ P.T._____ O.T._____ S.T. _____ MSS_____

Orders for Treatment:

Equipment:

Allergies:
Medications:

Home Care Coordinator _____

Date of Consult Request _____

1st Visit Made By _____

Primary Nurse _____

202-88

Figure B.1. Patient Referral Form

VISITING NURSE AND COMMUNITY HEALTH SERVICES
MEDICATION RECORD

PATIENT: CHART#:

ALLERGIES:

DATE/ INITIALS	MEDICATION	DOSAGE	FREQ	ROUTE USED	PURPOSE-EXPECTED SIDE EFFECTS	DATE	
						BEGUN	D/C

INITIALS	SIGNATURE/TITLE	INITIALS	SIGNATURE/TITLE

201-88

Figure B.2. Visiting Nurse and Community Health Services Medication Record

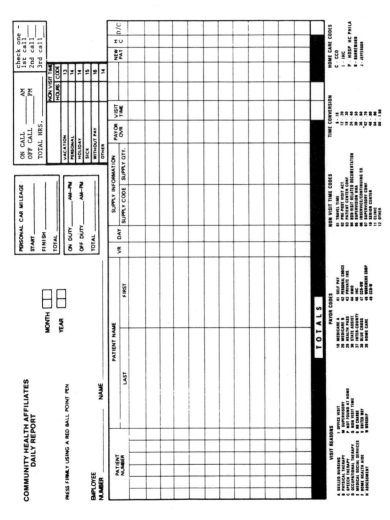

Figure B.3. Community Health Affiliates Daily Report

165

Supervisor Review:_____(initials)
                        _____(date)

COMMUNITY HEALTH AFFILIATES
CERTIFICATION AND PLAN OF CARE WORKSHEET (485)

Date _____ Employee Name_____ Employee# _____
New Patient _____ Recent/Change _____ Disciplines Ordered: Circle: SN   PT   ST   OT   MSS   Aide
Patient # _____ Patient Name _____ Payor _____ SOC_____-____-_____
Principal DX: Onset _____-_____-_____ ICD-9-Cm _____:_____:_____._____ Dx _____
Surgical Procedures: Onset _____-_____-_____ ICD-9-CM _____:_____:_____._____ Dx _____
Pertinent Dx: Onset _____-_____-_____ ICD-9-CM _____:_____:_____. DX _____
Other Pertinent DX: Onset _____-_____-_____ ICD-9-CM _____:_____:_____._____ Dx _____
Certification Date: From _____-_____-_____ To: _____-_____-_____

10. Medications (cross out if medication is discontinued)	Amt./Meas. dose	Freq. Code	Route Code	(N) (C)
Medications				

Dose: Amt of Measurement		Frequency Code:		Route Code:	
gm	gr	for additional codes	Q2H	Q0D	CL = Clysis	OD = right eye
ml	oz	last character must	Q3H	Q6W	EN = Ear/Nose	OS = left eye
cc	mg	be a letter	Q4H	QM	IM = Intramuscular	OU = Both eyes
puff			QID	PC	IVC = Intravenous Central	
			TID	AC	IVP = Intravenous Perip	
TSP	Teaspoon		BID	HS	OP = Opthalmis	
TBS	Tablespoon		qAM	QD	PO = Oral	
MEQ	gtt	unt-unit	qPM	QW	SQ = Subcutaneous	
MCG	tab	inc-inch		PRN	TO = Topical	
					PR = Per Rectum	
					VG = Vaginal	

For additional codes last
character must be: SL = Sublingual
H-Hr   IN = Inhale
D-Day   M-Month   NG = NG Tub/Gas
W-Week   ☐ See Addendum

Figure B.4. Community Health Affiliates Certification and Plan of Care Worksheet (485)

14. Medical Supplies & DME (ordered whether or not we supply them)

			Other
☐ 1. Dressing supplies	☐ 7. Cane	☐ 13. Commode	
☐ 2. Catheter supplies	☐ 8. Walker	☐ 14. Glucometer	_____
☐ 3. Ostomy supplies	☐ 9. Quadcane	☐ 15. Alt. Air Pressure	_____
☐ 4. Sterile solutions	☐ 10. Hospital Bed	Mattress	_____
☐ 5. Tube feeding supplies	☐ 11. Wheelchair		_____
☐ 6. O2	☐ 12. Siderails		

15. Safety Measures: all that apply

☐ 1. No Bending	☐ 5. Transfer with assist.	☐ 9. Restricted ROM	☐ 13. Activity superv.
☐ 2. No straining	☐ 6. No ambulation w/o assist.	☐ 10. No stairs	☐ 14. Oxygen precaution
☐ 3. No lifting	☐ 7. Remove environ. barriers	☐ 11. Attend at all times	☐ 15. Bedrails
☐ 4. No reaching	☐ 8. Amb. c assist device	☐ 12. Posey while OOB	☐ 16. Aspiration precautions

Other: _____

16. Nutritional Requirements: all that apply

☐ 1. Regular	☐ 6. Low Sodium	☐ 11. 1400 cal	☐ 16. Hi fiber	☐ 20. No conc. sweets
☐ 2. Soft	☐ 7. 2 gm Na	☐ 12. 1500 cal	☐ 17. Low fiber	☐ 21. Fluid restriction_____mls
☐ 3. Full liquid	☐ 8. 4 gm Na	☐ 13. 1800 cal	☐ 18. Hi calorie	☐ Other _____
☐ 4. Puree	☐ 9. 1000 cal	☐ 14. Diabetic	☐ 19. Hi protein	_____
☐ 5. Bland	☐ 10. 1200 cal	☐ 15. Low cholest.		_____

17. Allergies (medicine, food, etc.)

☐ NKA

18. A-Functional Limitations

☐ 1. Amputation	☐ 9. Legally blind
☐ 2. Bowel/Bladder (incont)	☐ A Dyspnea w/min. exertion
☐ 3. Contracture	☐ B Other (specify)
☐ 4. Hearing	☐ C Weakness
☐ 5. Paralysis	☐ D Swallowing
☐ 6. Endurance	☐ E Dependent ADLs
☐ 7. Ambulation	☐ F Paresis
☐ 8. Speech	☐ G Severe pain
B. Other _____	

18. B-Activities Permitted

☐ 1. Complete bedrest	☐ 9. Cane
☐ 2. Bedrest BRP	☐ A Wheelchair
☐ 3. Up to tolerated	☐ B Walker
☐ 4. Transfer bed/chair	☐ C No restrictions
☐ 5. Exercises prescribed .	☐ D Other (Specify)
☐ 6. Partial weight bearing	☐ H Hoyer lift transfers
☐ 7. Reserved	☐ J Amb. c assistance
☐ 8. Crutches	
D. Other _____	

19. Mental Status:

☐ 1. Oriented	☐ 3. Forgetful	☐ 5. Disoriented	☐ 7. Agitated
☐ 2. Comatose	☐ 4. Depressed	☐ 6. Lethargic	☐ 8. Other

20. Prognosis ☐ 1. Poor ☐ 2. Guarded ☐ 3. Fair ☐ 4. Good ☐ 5. Excellent

Figure B.4. Continued

Orders for discipline and treatment. Specify amount, frequency, duration. Include all disciplines and treatments, even if not billable to Medicare.

(Bold codes are Medicare used codes which may be transferred to 486)

Skilled nursing	Freq/Dur
☐ **A 0 Skilled Nursing** _____	___/___
☐ **A 1 Skilled Observation and Assessment of** ___	___/___
☐ _____	___/___
☐ _____	___/___

A100 Assess:

	Freq/Dur
☐ **A 33 ADL Status**	___/___
☐ **A 34 Mental Status**	___/___
☐ **A 35 Nutri. Status and Knowledge of Diet**	___/___
☐ **A 36 Body Weight/Fluid Balance**	___/___
☐ **A 37 Psychosocial Adjustment**	___/___
☐ **A 38 Skin Integrity**	___/___
☐ **A 39 For Referral to Therapies/MSS**	___/___
☐ **A 40 Edema**	___/___
☐ **A 41 S/S Hypoxia**	___/___
☐ **A 42 Pain Control**	___/___
☐ **A 43 Wound Healing**	___/___
☐ **A 44 Secretion Management**	___/___
☐ **A 45 Mechanical Ventilation**	___/___
☐ **A 46 Neuro Status**	___/___
☐ **A 47 Chemstrip/Blood Glucose Level**	___/___
☐ **A 48 Infant/Child Growth and Development**	___/___
☐ **A 49 Parent/Child Interaction**	___/___
☐ **A 50 Response to Medications**	___/___
☐ **A 51 Response to Chemotherapy**	___/___

Direct Care:

	Freq/Dur
☐ **A 2 Foley Insertion**	___/___
PRN up to _____ times for emergency irrigation and or catheter changes &/or assessment	
☐ **A3a** Bladder Instillation	___/___
☐ **A3b** Bladder Irrigation	___/___
☐ **A4** Open Wound Care/Dressing	___/___
☐ **A 5 Decubitis Care (stages 3, 4, & 5)**	___/___
☐ **A 6 Venipuncture**	___/___
and PRN _____ times for emergency	
☐ **A 7 Restorative Nursing**	___/___
☐ **A 8 Post Cateract Care**	___/___
☐ **A 9 Bowel/Bladder Training**	___/___
☐ **A 10 Chest Physio (incl Postural Drainage)**	___/___
☐ **A 11 Adm of Vitamin B-12**	___/___
☐ **A 12 Prep/Adm Insulin**	___/___

Skilled nursing	Freq/Dur
☐ **A 13 Adm Other IM/subq.**	___/___
☐ **A 14 Adm IVs/Clysis**	___/___
☐ **A 17 Reinsert Nasogastric Tube**	___/___
☐ **A 21 Adm Care of Trach**	___/___
☐ **A 23 Adm Inhalation Rx**	___/___
☐ **A 26 Disimpaction/F.U. Enema**	___/___
☐ **A 28 Wound Care/Dressing (Closed surg. inc)**	___/___
☐ **A 29 Decubitus Care (stage 1 & 2)**	___/___
☐ **A 53 Adm Chemo Therapy**	___/___
☐ **A 54 Adm CV Catheter Care**	___/___
☐ **A 55 Adm Infusaport Care**	___/___
☐ **A 56 Adm Care Biliary Drainage**	___/___
☐ **A 57 Adm Enema of Choice**	___/___
☐ **A 58 Reinsert Gastrostomy Tube**	___/___
☐ **A 59 Irrigate Hichman/Broviac Catheter**	___/___

A200 Teach:

	Freq/Dur
☐ **A 15 Ostomy/Illeoconduit Care**	___/___
☐ **A 16 Nasogastric Feeding**	___/___
☐ **A 18 Gastrostomy Feeding**	___/___
☐ **A 19 Patental Nutrition**	___/___
☐ **A 20 Care of Trach**	___/___
☐ **A 22 Inhalation Rx**	___/___
☐ **A 24 Adm of Injection**	___/___
☐ **A 25 Diabetic Care**	___/___
☐ **A 30 Care of Indwelling Catheter** (type of catheter _____).	___/___
☐ **A 32 Teach and Training**	___/___
☐ **A 60 Oxygen Therapy (__ l/ min. via ___)**	___/___
☐ **A 61 Special Equipment**	___/___
☐ **A 62 Special Procedure** _____	___/___
☐ **A 63 Suction**	___/___
☐ **A 64 Meds**	___/___
☐ **A 65 Diet**	___/___
☐ **A 66 Anticoagulant Precautions**	___/___
☐ **A 67 Aspiration Precautions**	___/___
☐ **A 68 Orthostatic Hypotension Precautions**	___/___
☐ **A 69 Energy Conservation**	___/___
☐ **A 70 Medical Emergency Procedures**	___/___
☐ **A 71 Blood Glucose Monitoring**	___/___
☐ **A 72 TED Hose Application**	___/___

Figure B.4. Continued

☐ A 73 Hickman Cath Care _____/_____
☐ A 74 Dressing Change Technique _____/_____
☐ A 75 Pumps _____/_____
☐ A 76 Skin Care _____/_____
☐ A 77 Ventilation Use _____/_____
☐ A 78 Breathing Exercises _____/_____
- -

A 27 Other (Specify) _____/_____
☐ **A 27** _____/_____
☐ **A 27** _____/_____
☐ **A 27** _____/_____
☐ **A 27** _____/_____
☐ **A 31** Mgmt and Eval of Pt. Care Plan _____/_____
☐ **A 79** Supervise Aide q 2 weeks _____/_____
- -

A 300 Notify
☐ A 80 MD of VS Abnormalities _____/_____
☐ A 81 MD of Med. Side Effects _____/_____
☐ A 82 MD of S/S Infection _____/_____
☐ A 83 MD of S/S Bleeding _____/_____
☐ A 84 MD of S/S Deterioration _____/_____
☐ A 85 MD of Wt. Gain above_____Lbs. _____/_____
☐ A 86 MD of (specify) _____
_____
_____

Home Health Aide   Freq/Dur
☐ F 0 Home Health Aide to Visit _____/_____
☐ F 1 Tub/Shower Bath
☐ F 2 Partial/Complete Bed Bath
☐ F 4 Personal Care ☐ Shave ☐ Shampoo
☐ F 6 Catheter Care
☐ F 8 Assist with Ambulation
☐ F10 Exercises
☐ F11 Prepare Meal

☐ F12 Grocery Shop
☐ F13 Wash Clothes
☐ F14 Housekeeping
☐ F15 Other (specify)_____
☐ F16 Assistance with Dressing
☐ F17 Assistance with Skin Care
☐ F18 Transfer Bed/Wheelchair
☐ F19 Weigh

22. Goals / Rehabilitation Potential / Discharge Plans

Realistic Goals:
Client/family independent in ☐ 1 meds ☐ 2 diet
    ☐ 3 treatment regime
Healed ☐ 4 leg ulcers ☐ 5 decubiti ☐ 6 wound
    ☐ 7 _____
☐ 8 Achieve optimum level of cardiovascular status.
☐ 9 Client/family use equipment properly and safely.
☐ 10 Compliance with medication/diet
☐ 11 Demonstrates correct insulin preparation/
    administration
Demonstrates self-care ability for ☐ 12 dressing change
☐ 13 wound care ☐ 14 ostomy care ☐ 15 diabetic care
    ☐ 16_____
☐ 17 Lab values within normal / therapeutic range.
☐ 18 Improved respiratory tolerance with activity.
☐ 19 Maintain patency of Foley Catheter and decrease
    risk of UTI.
☐ 20 Relief of Pain.
☐ 21 Relief of pain and symptoms until death.
☐ 22 Family able to care for client.
☐ 23 Able to manage at home with support services.

☐ 24 Client and family understand and accept long-term
    program.
Stable ☐ 25 diabetic status ☐ 26 cardiovascular status
    ☐ 27 respiratory status
☐ 28 Partial return to pre-illness level of functioning.
☐ 29 Complete return to pre-illness level of functioning.
☐ 30 Achieve maximum functional level of rehabilitation
    program.
☐ 31 Independent with ADL.
Independence with transfers ☐ 32 complete ☐ 33 partial
Able to ambulate ☐ 34 with ☐ 35 without assistive
                                 device in_____weeks
☐ 36 Increased ROM of _____
☐ 37 Prosthetic ambulation with assistive device in
    _____weeks
Improved ☐ 38 balance ☐ 39 tone ☐ 40 coordination
☐ 41 Verbal expression is understandable.
☐ 42 Improved cognitive functioning.
☐ Other _____
_____

Figure B.4. Continued

COMMUNITY HEALTH AFFILIATES
NURSING MEDICAL UPDATE AND PATIENT INFORMATION WORKSHEET (486)

Patient's Name_____ #_____ Nurse_____

8. Medicare Covered Yes ☐ No ☐   9. Date Physician Last Saw Patient_____ 10. Date Last Contacted Dr._____

11. Is the Patient Receiving Care in an 1861 (J)(I) Skilled Nursing Facility or Equivalent ? Yes ☐ No ☐ Do Not Know ☐

12. Certification ☐ Recertification ☐ Modified ☐

13.   **Specific Services and Treatments**

Discipline	Visits (This bill) Ret. to Prior Cert.	Frequency and Duration	Treatment Codes	Total Visits Projected This Cert.
RN				
AIDE				

14. Dates of Last Inpatient Stay   15. Type of Facility ☐ 1. Hospital (acute)   ☐ 4. Nursing Home
      Admission _____   ☐ 2. Hospital (rehab)   ☐ 5. Other_____
      Discharge _____   ☐ 3. Skilled Nursing Unit   _____

16. UPDATE INFORMATION: New Orders / Treatments / Clinical Facts / Summary from Each Discipline (aides also)
Write the Discipline before starting the notation
Vital Signs: AP_____ RP_____ Resp_____ BP_____ Site_____ BP_____ Site_____ Temp_____

_____
_____
_____
_____
_____
_____
_____

17. Functional Limitations (Expand from 485 and Level of ADL):_____

_____

• Homebound Reason • (check all that apply)
☐ A Confused/disoriented/lacks judgment ☐ B Short of breath upon exertion ☐ C Bedbound
☐ D Unable to navigate stairs   ☐ E Needs considerable assistance of at least one other person to leave home
☐ F Sensory-neuro deficit   ☐ G Bed to chair/wheelchair   ☐ H Needs assistive device_____
☐ I Severely restricted ROM due to_____
☐ J Actively limited to instability of disease process   ☐ K Cardiac limitations ☐ L Impaired ambulation
☐ M Severe Pain   ☐ N_____
Prior Functional Status:_____
_____

18. Supplementary Plan of Treatment on File from Physician Other than Referring Physician: Yes ☐ No ☐
(If yes, please specify giving Goals/Rehab. Potential/Discharge Plan)_____

19. Unusual Home/Social Environment ☐ 1 NA ☐ 2 Lives Alone ☐ 3 Lives with impaired member of family ☐ 4 Other_____	21. Specify any known medical and/or nonmedical reasons the patient regularly leaves home and frequency of occurrence. ☐ 1 MD appointment approx. 30 to 60 days ☐ 2 Hospitalized—specify:_____ ☐ 3 Other_____
20. Indicate any time when the home health agency made a visit and patient was not home and reason if ascertainable	22. Nurse or therapist completing or reviewing form: Date (mo, day, yr)_____
P.T. Only—No Aide: Nurse Complete all except # 13, 16, 17, 18, & 19	P.T. Only with Aide: Nurse complete all except # 17 & 18

Figure B.5. Community Health Affiliates Nursing Medical Update and Patient Information Worksheet (486)

PHYSICAL THERAPY
CERTIFICATION AND PLAN OF CARE WORKSHEET (485)

Date _____ Employee Name_____ Employee# _____
New Patient _____ Recent/Change _____
Patient # _____ Patient Name _____ Payor _____ SOC____-___-__
Additional Diagnosis: Onset ____-___-____ ICD-9-Cm ____:____:___-____
Dx _____ Certification Date: From ____-___-__ To: ___-___-__
21. Orders for Discipline and Treatments—Specify Amount Frequency/Duration

PHYSICAL THERAPY

		Freq/Dur			Freq/Dur
			MUST be Checked with a Freq/Dur		
__B0	Physical Therapy Freq/Dur	__/__	__B10	Fabrication of Temporary Devices	__/__
__B1	Evaluation	__/__	__B18	Active Exercise	__/__
__B2	Therapeutic exercise	__/__	__B19	Resistive Exercise	__/__
__B3	Transfer Training	__/__	__B20	Stretching Exercises	__/__
__B4	Home Program	__/__	__B9	Prosthetic Training	__/__
__B5	Gait Training	__/__	__B21	Whirlpool***	__/__
__B16(A)	Proprioceptive Neuromuscular Facilitation		__B7	Ultrasound	__/__
			__B22	Coordination Exercises	__/__
__B6	Chest Physiotherapy	__/__	__B8	Electro-Therapy	__/__
__B17	Passive Exercises	__/__	__B23	Therapeutic Heat/Cold	__/__
__B15	Other (specify orders)	__/__	__B11	Muscle Re-education	__/__
			__B25	Supervise HHA q 2 weeks	__/__
			__B12	Management and Evaluation	__/__

22. Goals/Rehabilitation Potential / Discharge Plans

Realistic Goals:
Client/family independent in ☐ 1 meds ☐ 2 diet
   ☐ 3 treatment regime
Healed ☐ 4 leg ulcers ☐ 5 decubiti ☐ 6 wound
   ☐ 7 _____
☐ 8 Achieve optimum level of cardiovascular status.
☐ 9 Client/family use equipment properly and safely.
☐ 10 Compliance with medication/diet.
☐ 11 Demonstrates correct insulin preparation/
   administration.
Demonstrates self-care ability for ☐ 12 dressing change
☐ 13 wound care ☐ 14 ostomy care ☐ 15 diabetic care
☐ 16 _____
☐ 17 Lab values within normal / therapeutic range.
☐ 18 Improved respiratory tolerance with activity.
☐ 19 Maintain patency of Foley Catheter and decrease in
   risk of UTI.
☐ 20 Relief of Pain.
☐ 21 Relief of pain and symptoms until death.
☐ 22 Family able to care for client.
☐ 23 Able to manage at home with support services.

☐ 24 Client and family understand and accept long term
   program.
Stable ☐ 25 diabetic status ☐ 26 cardiovascular status
   ☐ 27 respiratory status
☐ 28 Partial return to pre-illness level of functioning.
☐ 29 Complete return to pre-illness level of functioning.
☐ 30 Achieve maximum functional level of rehabilitation
   program.
☐ 31 Independent with ADL.
Independence with transfers ☐ 32 complete ☐ 33 partial
Able to ambulate ☐ 34 with ☐ 35 without assistive device
   in _____weeks
☐ 36 Increased ROM of _____
☐ 37 Prosthetic ambulation with assistive device in
   _____weeks
Improved ☐ 38 balance ☐ 39 tone ☐ 40 coordination
☐ 41 Verbal expression is understandable.
☐ 42 Improved cognitive functioning.
☐ Other _____

Figure B.6. Physical Therapy Certification and Plan of Care Worksheet (485)

Rehabilitation Potential:
Write on the line for the "potential" **G** Good **F** Fair **P** Poor
Rehab potential
__ ☐ 1 for achieving goals.
__ ☐ for stable ☐ 2 diabetic status ☐ 3 BP ☐ 4 cardiac status
__ ☐ 5 respiratory ☐ 6_____
__ ☐ for ☐ 7 self-management ☐ 8 family management of dis-
            ease entity
__ ☐ for improved ☐ 9 nutritional status ☐ 10 respiratory status
__ ☐ 11 cardiac status
__ ☐ for ☐ 12 self care ☐ 13 catheter change ☐ 12 B-12
                                                    injection
__ ☐ 15 _____may always be needed.
__ ☐ for ☐ 16 partial ☐ 17 complete return to pre-illness level
                    of functioning.
__ ☐ 18 for achieving maximum functional level with rehab.
        program.
__ for return to independent ambulation ☐ 19 with
__ ☐ 20 w/out assistive device.
__ ☐ 21 for return to independence in ADLs.
__ ☐ 22 for increased activity tolerance.
__ ☐ 23 client ☐ 24 family learning use of equipment.
__ ☐ 25 understandable speech.
__ ☐ 26 use of alternative communication system.
__ ☐ _____
    _____

Diacharge Plan:

__ Discharge to ☐ 50 self care ☐ 51 family care
☐ 52 family and self care ☐ 53 hired caregiver
__ 54 Referral for out-patient care when no longer home bound.
__ 55 Referral for support services when skilled care is no
     longer needed.
☐ 56 Home health care will be needed until admission to nursing
     home or death.
__ Will always need assistance with ☐ 57 ADL.
☐ 58 Ambulation ☐ 59 Ostomy care ☐ _____
__ 60 Will need terminal care until client expires.

Write out if applicable

For daily care (5-7 days) write the goal and expected end date:

23. Verbal SOC date

    Date VO received for first visit_____from Dr._____

                    —OR—

    Date VO received to continue services _____from Dr._____

    Nurse Signature_____Date_____

24. Physician Name_____Phone_____

    Address_____

Figure B.6. Continued

COMMUNITY HEALTH AFFILIATES
MEDICAL UPDATE AND PATIENT INFORMATION WORKSHEET (486)

DISCIPLINE (Circle One) P.T. O.T. S.T. M.S.S.

Patient's Name_____#_____Therapist/S.W._____

13. **Specific Services and Treatments**

Discipline	Visits (This Bill) Rel. to Prior Cert.	Frequency and Duration	Treatment Codes	Total Visits Projected This Cert.
PT				
ST				
OT				
MSS				
Aide				

16. UPDATE INFORMATION: New Orders / Treatments / Clinical Facts / Summary from Each Discipline (aides also)
Write the Discipline before starting the notation.
Vital Signs AP_____ RP_____ Resp_____ BP_____ Site_____ BP_____ Site_____ Temp_____

_____
_____
_____
_____
_____
_____
_____

17. Functional Limitations (Expand from 485 and Level of ADL); Reason Homebound / Prior Functional Status

_____

Check all that apply:
☐ A Confused/disoriented/lacks judgment ☐ B Short of breath upon exertion ☐ C Bedbound
☐ D Unable to navigate stairs ☐ E Needs considerable assistance of at least one other person to leave home
☐ F Sensory-neuro deficit ☐ G Bed to chair/wheelchair ☐ H Needs assistive device_____
☐ I Severely restricted ROM due to_____
☐ J Actively limited to instability of disease process ☐ K Cardiac limitations ☐ L Impaired ambulation
☐ M Severe Pain ☐ N_____

18. Supplementary Plan of Treatment on File from Physician Other than Referring Physician: Yes☐ No ☐
If yes, please specify giving Goals /Rehab. Potential /Discharge Plan_____

19. Unusual Home/Social Environment
☐ 1 NA
☐ 2 Lives alone
☐ 3 Lives with impaired member of family
☐ 4 Other_____

22. Nurse or therapist completing or reviewing form:
_____ _____
Date (mo, day, yr)_____

Figure B.7. Community Health Affiliates Medical Update and Patient Information Worksheet (486)

SPEECH THERAPY
CERTIFICATION AND PLAN OF CARE WORKSHEET (485)

Date _____ Employee Name_____ Employee# _____
New Patient _____ Recent/Change _____
Patient # _____ Patient Name _____ Payor _____ SOC_____-____-_____
Additional Diagnosis: Onset _____-_____-_____ ICD-9-Cm _____:_____:_____
Dx _____ Certification Date: From _____-_____-_____ To: _____-_____-_____
21. Orders for Discipline and Treatments-Specify Amount Frequency/Duration

SPEECH THERAPY

		Freq/Dur			Freq/Dur
			Must be Checked with a Freq/Dur		
__C0	Speech Therapy Freq/Dur	____/____	__C13	Retraining Written Communication	____/____
__C1	Evaluation	____/____	__C14	Retraining Reading Communication	____/____
__C10	Alaryngeal Speech	____/____			
__C5	Language Disorders Treatment	____/____	__C2	Voice Disorders Treatment	____/____
__C11	Comprehensive	____/____	__C3(A)	Speech Articulation Disorders Rx	____/____
__C6	Aural Rehabilitation	____/____			
__C12	Aug. Com. Training	____/____	__C15	Retraining Oral-Motor Patterns	____/____
__C4	Dysphagia Therapy and Education	____/____	__C16	Verbal Expression	____/____
			__C8	Non-Oral Communication	____/____
__C9	Other (Specify Orders)	____/____	__C9	Other (Specify Orders)	____/____

22. Goals / Rehabilitation Potential / Discharge Plans

Realistic Goals:
Client/family independent in ☐ 1 meds ☐ 2 diet
  ☐ 3 treatment regime
Healed ☐ 4 leg ulcers ☐ 5 decubiti ☐ 6 wound
  ☐ 7 _____
☐ 8 Achieve optimum level of cardiovascular status.
☐ 9 Client/family use equipment properly and safely.
☐ 10 Compliance with medication/diet.
☐ 11 Demonstrates correct insulin preparation/
  administration.
Demonstrates self-care ability for ☐ 12 dressing change
☐ 13 wound care ☐ 14 ostomy care ☐ 15 diabetic care
☐ 16 _____
☐ 17 Lab values within normal/therapeutic range.
☐ 18 Improved respiratory tolerance with activity.
☐ 19 Maintain patency of Foley Catheter and decrease in
  risk of UTI.
☐ 20 Relief of Pain.
☐ 21 Relief of pain and symptoms until death.
☐ 22 Family able to care for client.
☐ 23 Able to manage at home with support services.

☐ 24 Client and family understand and accept long-term
  program.
Stable ☐ 25 diabetic status ☐ 26 cardiovascular status
  ☐ 27 respiratory status
☐ 28 Partial return to pre-illness level of functioning.
☐ 29 Complete return to pre-illness level of functioning.
☐ 30 Achieve maximum functional level of rehabilitation
  program.
☐ 31 Independent with ADL.
Independence with transfers ☐ 32 complete ☐ 33 partial
Able to ambulate ☐ 34 with ☐ 35 without assistive device
  in _____ weeks
☐ 36 Increased ROM of _____
☐ 37 Prosthetic ambulation with assistive device in
  _____ weeks.
Improved ☐ 38 balance ☐ 39 tone ☐ 40 coordination
☐ 41 Verbal expression is understandable.
☐ 42 Improved cognitive functioning.
☐ Other _____
  _____

Figure B.8. Speech Therapy Certification and Plan of Care Worksheet (485)

OCCUPATIONAL THERAPY
CERTIFICATION AND PLAN OF CARE WORKSHEET (485)

Date _____ Employee Name_____ Employee # _____
New Patient _____ Recent/Change _____ __
Patient # _____ Patient Name _____ Payor _____ SOC_____-____-_____
Additional Diagnosis: Onset _____-_____-_____ ICD-9-Cm _____:_____:_____.____
Dx _____ Certification Date: From _____-_____-_____ To: _____-_____-_____
21. Orders for Discipline and Treatments - Specify Amount Frequency/Duration

OCCUPATIONAL THERAPY

		Freq/Dur			Freq/Dur
				Must be Checked with a Freq/Dur	
__D0	Occupational Therapy		__D18	Instruction in Transfers	___/___
	Freq/Dur. _____		__D19	Instruction in Cooking	___/___
__D1	Evaluation	___/___	__D20	Inst. in Homemaking /House-	___/___
__D2	Independent Living-Daily Skills	___/___		keeping	
__D3	Muscle Re-Education	___/___	__D6	Fine Motor Coordination	___/___
__D12	Ther. EX to UE	___/___	__D21	Act. To Increase Writing	___/___
__D13	Ex. To Increase UE Strength	___/___		Ability	
__D14	Ex. to improve Self Care	___/___	__D15	Instruction in Dressing	___/___
__D22	Reality Orientation Ex.	___/___	__D16	Instruction in Grooming	___/___
__D23	Ex. to Improve Abstract	___/___	__D17	Instruction in Bathing	___/___
	Reasoning		__D5	Perceptual Motor Training	___/___
__D4	Reserved	___/___	__D9	Orthotics/Splinting	___/___
__D8	Sensory Treatment	___/___	__D10	Adaptive Equiptment	___/___
__D7	Neuro-Development Rx	___/___	__D11	Other (Specify Orders)	___/___
__D11	Other (Specify Orders)	___/___		_____	
				_____	

22. Goals/Rehabilitation Potential / Discharge Plans

Realistic Goals:
Client/family independent in ☐ 1 meds ☐ 2 diet
   ☐ 3 treatment regime
Healed ☐ 4 leg ulcers ☐ 5 decubiti ☐ 6 wound
  ☐ 7 _____
☐ 8 Achieve optimum level of cardiovascular status.
☐ 9 Client/family use equipment properly and safely.
☐ 10 Compliance with medication/diet.
☐ 11 Demonstrates correct insulin preparation/
   administration.
Demonstrations self-care ability for ☐ 12 dressing change
☐ 13 wound care ☐ 14 ostomy care ☐ 15 diabetic care
☐ 16 _____
☐ 17 Lab values within normal / therapeutic range.
☐ 18 Improved respiratory tolerance with activity.
☐ 19 Maintain patency of Foley Catheter and decrease in
   risk of UTI
☐ 20 Relief of pain.
☐ 21 Relief of pain and symptoms until death.
☐ 22 Family able to care for client.
☐ 23 Able to manage at home with support services.

☐ 24 Client and family understand and accept long term
   program.
Stable ☐ 25 diabetic status ☐ 26 cardiovascular status
   ☐ 27 respiratory status
☐ 28 Partial return to pre-illness level of functioning.
☐ 29 Complete return to pre-illness level of functioning.
☐ 30 Achieve maximum functional level of rehabilitation
   program.
☐ 31 Independent with ADL.
Independence with transfers ☐ 32 complete ☐ 33 partial
Able to ambulate ☐ 34 with ☐ 35 without assistive device
               in _____ weeks
☐ 36 Increased ROM of _____
☐ 37 Prosthetic ambulation with assistive device in
     _____ weeks
Improved ☐ 38 balance ☐ 39 tone ☐ 40 coordination
☐ 41 Verbal expression is understandable.
☐ 42 Improved cognitive functioning.
☐ Other _____

Figure B.10. Occupational Therapy Certification and Plan of Care Worksheet (485)

MEDICAL SOCIAL SERVICES
CERTIFICATION AND PLAN OF CARE WORKSHEET (485)

Date _____ Employee Name_____ Employee # _____

New Patient _____ Recent/Change _____

Patient # _____ Patient Name _____ Payor _____ SOC_____-____-_____

Additional Diagnosis: Onset _____-_____-_____ ICD-9-Cm _____:_____:_____-_____

Dx _____ Certification Date: From _____-_____-_____ To: _____-_____-_____

21. Orders for Discipline and Treatments - Specify Amount Frequency/Duration

MEDICAL SOCIAL SERVICES

Must be Checked with a Freq/Dur

___E0	Medical Social Services		
	Freq/Dur._____	___E17	Evaluation & Assessment of Chemical
___E1	Assessment of Social and Emotional	___E17A	Abuse or Dependency (Drug or Alcohol)
___E1A	Factors		
___E	Counseling Adjustment to Illness	___E18	Referrals to Appropriate Inpatient/Out
___E7	Counseling Family/Caregiver	___E18A	Patient Services for Chemical Abuse or
___E8	Financial Assistant with	___E18B	Dependency
___E8A	Budgeting		
___E9	Placement Assistance	___E19	Assist with Relocation
___E10	Arrange for Meals	___E20	Assessment and Evaluation of
___E11	Terminal Illness Counseling	___E20A	Adult/Abuse/Neglect
___E12	Counseling for Linkage to Ongoing	___E21	Referrals to Appropriate Agencies to
___E12A	Services		
___E13	Assistance with Linkage to Community	___E21A	Intervene in Potential or Ongoing Adult
___E13A	Agencies Dealing with Financial Needs	___E21B	Abuse
___E	Arrange Transportation	___E14	Explanation of Insurance Benefits
___E16	Assessment of Home Situation	___E15	Assess/Child Abuse/Neglect
___E2	Counseling for Long Range Planning and	___E4	Short Term Therapy
___E2A	Decision Making	___E5	Reserved
___E6	Other (Specify Orders)	___E3	Community Resource Planning

Some of the above codes need to use 2 or 3 codes to have the full description appear

E1   Entered as E1, E1A
E2   Entered as E2, E2A
E12   Entered as E12, E12A,
E13   Entered as E13, E13A
E17   Entered as E17, E17A
E18   Entered as E18, E18A, E18B
E20   Entered as E20, E20A
E21   Entered as E21, E21A, E21B

Figure B.12. Medical Social Services Certification and Plan of Care Worksheet (485)

22. Goals/Rehabilitation Potential / Discharge Plans

Realistic Goals:

Client/family independent in ☐ 1 meds ☐ 2 diet
   ☐ 3 treatment regime
Healed ☐ 4 leg ulcers ☐ 5 decubiti ☐ 6 wound
   ☐ 7 _____
☐ 8 Achieve optimum level of cardiovascular status.
☐ 9 Client/family use equipment properly and safely.
☐ 10 Compliance with medication/diet.
☐ 11 Demonstrates correct insulin preparation/
   administration.
Demonstrates self-care ability for ☐ 12 dressing change
☐ 13 wound care ☐ 14 ostomy care ☐ 15 diabetic care
☐ 16 _____
☐ 17 Lab values within normal/therapeutic range.
☐ 18 Improved respiratory tolerance with activity.
☐ 19 Maintain patency of Foley Catheter and decrease in
   risk of UTI.
☐ 20 Relief of Pain.
☐ 21 Relief of pain and symptoms until death.
☐ 22 Family able to care for client.
☐ 23 Able to manage at home with support services.

☐ 24 Client and family understand and accept long-term
   program.
Stable ☐ 25 diabetic status ☐ 26 cardiovascular status
   ☐ 27 respiratory status.
☐ 28 Partial return to pre-illness level of functioning.
☐ 29 Complete return to pre-illness level of functioning.
☐ 30 Achieve maximum functional level of rehabilitation
   program.
☐ 31 Independent with ADL.
Independence with transfers ☐ 32 complete ☐ 33 partial
Able to ambulate ☐ 34 with ☐ 35 without assistive device
   in _____ weeks
☐ 36 Increased ROM of _____
☐ 37 Prosthetic ambulation with assistive device in
   _____ weeks.
Improved ☐ 38 balance ☐ 39 tone ☐ 40 coordination
☐ 41 Verbal expression is understandable.
☐ 42 Improved cognitive functioning.
☐ Other _____
_____

Rehabilitation Potential:
Write on the line for the "potential" G Good F Fair P Poor
Rehab potential
__ ☐ 1 for achieving goals
__ ☐ for stable ☐ 2 diabetic status ☐ 3 BP ☐ 4 cardiac status
__ ☐ 5 respiratory ☐ 6 _____
__ ☐ for ☐ 7 self-management ☐ 8 family management of
           disease entity
__ ☐ for improved ☐ 9 nutritional status ☐ 10 respiratory status
__ ☐ 11 cardiac status
__ ☐ for ☐ 12 self care ☐ 13 catheter change ☐ 12 B-12
                    injection
__ ☐ 15 _____ may always be needed.
__ ☐ for ☐ 16 partial ☐ 17 complete return to pre-illness level
           functioning.
__ ☐ 18 for achieving maximum functional level with rehab.
   program.
____ for return to independent ambulation ☐ 19 with
__ ☐ 20 w/out assistive device.
__ ☐ 21 for return to independence in ADLs.
__ ☐ 22 for increased activity tolerance.
__ ☐ 23 Client ☐ 24 family learning use of equipment.
__ ☐ 25 understandable speech.
__ ☐ 26 use of alternative communication system.
__ ☐ _____

Discharge Plan:

__ Discharge to ☐ 50 self care ☐ 51 family care
☐ 52 family and self care ☐ 53 hired caregiver
__ 54 Referral for out-patient care when no longer home bound.
__ 55 Referral for support services when skilled care is no longer
   needed.
__ 56 Home health care will be needed until admission to nursing home or death.
__ Will always need assistance with ☐ 57 ADL.
☐ 58 Ambulation ☐ 59 Ostomy care ☐ _____
__ 60 Will need terminal care until client expires.

Write out if applicable

For daily care (5-7 days) write the goal and expected end date:

Figure B.12. Continued

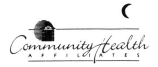

PATIENT AGREEMENT FOR TREATMENT AND RELEASE OF INFORMATION

This Agreement is entered into by and between Visiting Nurse and Community Health Services (hereinafter called Agency) and _____ (hereinafter called Patient.)

In consideration of the service to be provided by the Agency, it is agreed as follows:

1. **TREATMENT AUTHORIZATION:** In the knowledge that my state of health requires the services of the Agency, I voluntarily consent and agree to actively participate in such services as assessments, treatments, personal care and therapeutic exercises prescribed by my physician and rendered by Nurses, Physical Therapists, Occupational Therapists, Speech Pathologists, Social Workers and Home Health Aides. I understand that the Agency has specific policies relating to the care provided to me and these policies include provision for termination of services at my request, request of physician and/or decision of the Agency. I agree to abide by the terms of these Agency policies in all respects.

2. **NON-DISCRIMINATON:** Agency and Patient hereby agree that services are rendered without regard to race, color, sex, age or national origin.

3. **RELEASE OF INFORMATION:** I authorize the Agency to furnish information from my records to any of my insurers and to all other agencies, institutions, or individuals providing health or social services to me. Consent is also given for the release of information to the Agency by any insurer and all other agencies, institutions or individuals from whom I have received medical or social services. Consent is also given for the release of information in a summary or statistical form which does not identify particular individuals.

4. **SOCIAL SECURITY ACT, TITLE XVIII (MEDICARE):** I understand that application for payment under Title XVIII of the Social Security Act may be made, and that information need be given by Patient in order to receive such payment. I certify that the information given by Patient in applying for payment under Title XVIII of the Social Security Act is correct. I request that payment of authorized Medicare benefits be made for and on Patient's behalf.

5. **AUTHORIZATION TO PAY INSURANCE BENEFITS:** I authorize payment of benefits directly to the Agency for credit to my account. I understand that I will be notified of any such payments made to the Agency as provider of service and that I am financially responsible to the Agency for charges not covered by my insurance benefits.

I, the undersigned, have read, understood and received a copy of this agreement on _____
                                                                                                    (Date)

Patient Signature _____   If patient signs by "X":

Address _____   Witness _____
          _____   _____ Agency Representative
                                                              _____ Relative/Responsible Party
                                                                       Specify relationship: _____
                                                                       _____

Reason patient did not sign or used "X": _____ Minor _____ Physically Unable _____ Mentally Unable

Responsible Party Signature _____

Address _____

Relationship to Patient _____

Figure B.14. Patient Agreement for Treatment and Release of Information

Community Health
A F F I L I A T E S
104-108 Ardmore Avenue
Ardmore, Pennsylvania 19003

PLAN OF CARE
HOME HEALTH AIDE

PATIENT'S NAME		PATIENT I.D. NO.	
ADDRESS		PHONE NO.	
	D.O.B.	FEE SOURCE	
RESPONSIBLE PERSON		PHONE NO.	
PRIMARY NURSE		PHONE NO.	
PRIMARY AIDE		FREQUENCY	HOURS

SERVICES TO BE PERFORMED: (CHECK THOSE WHICH APPLY)

SERVICES	COMMENTS	SERVICES	COMMENTS
☐ BATHING		☐ FORCE FLUIDS	
☐ BED		☐ FEEDING	
☐ TUB		☐ MEAL PREPARATION	
☐ SHOWER		☐ POSITIONING	
☐ SPONGE		☐ TURNING	
☐ SPECIAL SKIN CARE		☐ PASSIVE RANGE OF MOTION	
☐ ORAL HYGIENE		☐ TRANSFER	
☐ NAIL CARE		☐ AMBULATION	
☐ FOOT CARE		☐ CHG. BED LINENS	
☐ TOILETING		☐ PERSONAL LAUND.	
☐ SHAVING		☐ OTHER (Specify)	
☐ DRESSING			
☐ INTAK/OUTPUT			

GOAL: _____ DISCHARGE PLAN: _____

EQUIPMENT: ☐ WHEELCHAIR ☐ WALKER ☐ O_2 ☐ COMMODE ☐ HOSPITAL BED

ALLERGIES: _____

SAFETY MEASURES: _____

DATE OF REFERRAL _____ NURSES'S SIGNATURE _____

White - Patient's Record, Yellow - Home, Pink - Home Health Aide Agency CHSS Other:
(Indicate One)

403-88

Figure B.15. Plan of Care Home Health Aide

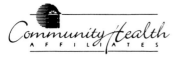 **PATIENT'S BILL OF RIGHTS**

Community Health Affiliates (CHA) protects and promotes your rights as a patient under its care.
You have:

1. The right to be fully informed in writing of your rights and responsibilities.

2. The right to be fully informed in advance about the care and treatment to be provided by
   CHA, and the changes in that care or treatment which may affect your well-being, as well as
   the right to participate in planning care and treatment or changes in same.

3. The right to proper identification, by name and title, of all personnel involved in your care.

4. The right to privacy and confidentiality.

5. The right to have all clinical records pertaining to your care treated as confidential, except
   as otherwise provided by law or third party reimbursement arrangements.

6. The right to refuse any treatment, procedure, or medication within the confines of the law,
   and to be informed of the consequences of doing so.

7. The right to receive medically appropriate services without discrimination based upon your
   race, color, religion, sex, age, or national origin.

8. The right to access, upon request, all information contained in your clinical record.

9. The right to know the procedure for voicing grievances and suggesting changes in service
   or staff without fear of restraint or discrimination.

10. The right to be informed of services available, charges for services, and eligibility for third
    party reimbursement.

11. The right to be informed of any changes in the services, charges, or eligibility for third party
    reimbursement.

12. The right to be informed in advance of anticipated termination of service or plans for
    transfer to another agency.

13. The right to be informed of the availability of the Pennsylvania state home health agency
    hotline to communicate unresolved problems:
    Medicare Beneficiaries Call:
    PENNSYLVANIA DEPARTMENT OF HEALTH   **1-800-222-0989**
    Division of Primary Care and Home Health Services

    In person response Monday through Friday from 8:30 a.m. to 5:00 p.m. After hours,
    weekends and holiday messages may be left on an answering machine for response
    the next working day.

    KEYSTONE PEER REVIEW ORGANIZATION   **1-800-322-1914**

    I hereby acknowledge receipt of the foregoing statement of my rights as a patient of
    Community Health Affiliates.

_____   _____   _____
Patient Signature   Witness Signature   Date

White – clinical record; Yellow – patient copy

Figure B.16. Patient's Bill of Rights

References

Ahmann, E. (1986). *Home care for the high risk infant: A holistic guide to using technology.* Frederick, MD: Aspen.

Aspen Reference Group. (1989). *Home health care—Forms, checklists & guidelines.* Gaithersburg, MD: Aspen.

Austin, M. J. (1981). *Supervisory management for the human services.* Englewood Cliffs, NJ: Prentice-Hall.

Axelrod, T. (1978, August). Innovative roles for social workers in home care programs. *Health and Social Work, 3*(3), 48-66.

Barbieri, E. B. (1983, March). Patient falls are not patient accidents. *Journal of Gerontological Nursing, 9*(3), 165-174.

Beland, F. (1984). The decision of elderly persons to leave their homes. *The Gerontologist, 24*(2), 179-185.

Boothe, W. H. (1986). Competition in home health care. In S. Stuart-Siddall (Ed.), *Home health care nursing: Administrative and clinical perspectives* (pp. 93-104). Rockville, MD: Aspen.

Branch, L. G., & Jette, A. M. (1983). Elders' use of informal long-term care assistance. *The Gerontologist, 23*(1), 51-56.

Brickner, P. W. (1978). *Home health care for the aged: How to help older people stay in their own homes and out of institutions.* New York: Appleton-Century-Crofts.

Brody, E. M. (1977). *Long-term care of older people.* New York: Human Sciences Press.

Browdie, R. B., & Turwoski, A. (1986). The problems of providing services to the elderly in their own homes. In A. O. Pelham & W. F. Clark (Eds.), *Managing home care for the elderly: Lessons from community-based agencies* (pp. 31-46). New York: Springer.

Buglass, K. (1989). The business of eldercare. *American Demographics, 11,* 32-39.

Bulau, J. M. (1986). *Clinical policies and procedures for home health care.* Rockville, MD: Aspen.

Bulau, J. M. (1991). *Administrative policies and procedures for home health care* (2nd ed.). Rockville, MD: Aspen.

Bumagin, V. E., & Hirn, K. F. (1990). *Helping the aging family: A guide for professionals.* Glenview, IL: Scott, Foresman and Company.

Burack-Weiss, A., & Brennan, F. C. (1984). *First encounters between elders and agencies: A practice guide.* New York: Brookdale Institute on Aging and Adult Human Development, Columbia University.

Cantor, M. H. (1985). Families: A basic source of long-term care for the elderly. *Aging, 349,* 8-13.

Caplan, G. (1961). *An approach to community mental health.* New York: Grune & Stratton.

Coile, Jr., R. C. (1990). Technology and ethics: Three scenarios for the 1990s. *Quality Review Bulletin, 16* 202-208.

Cooper, P. (Ed.). (1979). *Health care marketing.* Rockville, MD: Aspen.

Duke University, OARS. (1978). *Multidimensional functional assessment: The OARS methodology* (2nd ed.). Durham, NC: Center for the Study of Aging and Human Development, Duke University.

Fessler, S. R., & Adams, C. G. (1985). Nurse/social worker role conflict in home health care. *Journal of Gerontological Social Work, 9,* 113-123.

Fillenbaum, G. G. (1987). Multidimensional functional assessment. In G. L. Maddox (Ed.), *The encyclopedia of aging* (pp. 460-462). New York: Springer.

Fortinsky, R. H., Granger, C. V., & Seltzer, G. B. (1981, May). The use of functional assessment in understanding home care needs. *Medical Care, XIX*(5), 489-497.

Friedman, S. R., & Kaye, L. W. (1979). Homecare for the frail elderly: implications for an interactional relationship. *Journal of Gerontological Social Work, 2*(2), 109-123.

Garner, D. J., & Mercer, S. O. (1982). Meeting the needs of the elderly: Home health care or institutionalization? *Health and Social Work, 7*(3), 183-191.

Gilbertson, E. (1981). *A better answer: Homemaker-home health aide services for persons with developmental disabilities and their families.* New York: National HomeCaring Council.

Gilroy, P., Trager, B., & Kinney, T. (1982). *Supervision in home care: A manual for supervisors.* Washington, DC: National HomeCaring Council.

Ginzberg, E., Balinsky, W., & Ostow, M. (1984). *Home health care: Its role in the changing health services market.* Totowa, NJ: Rowman & Allanheld.

Glosser, G., Wexler, D., & Balmelli, M. (1985). Physicians' and families' perspectives on the medical management of dementia. *Journal of the American Geriatrics Society, 33,* 383-391.

Gould, E. J., & Wargo, J. (1987). *Home health nursing care plans.* Rockville, MD: Aspen.

Gurland, B. J., & Wilder, D. E. (1984). The CARE interview revisited: Development of an efficient, systematic, clinical assessment. *Journal of Gerontology, 39,* 129-137.

Haddad, A. M. (1987). *High tech home care: A practical guide.* Rockville, MD: Aspen.

Hastings Center. (1987). *Guidelines on the termination of life sustaining treatment and the care of the dying.* Bloomington: Indiana University Press.

Herr, J. J., & Weakland, J. H. (1979). *Counseling elders and their families: Practical techniques for applied gerontology.* New York: Springer.

Hodgson, J. H., & Quinn, J. L. (1980). The impact of the triage health care delivery system upon client morale, independent living, and the cost of care. *The Gerontologist, 20*(3), 364-371.

Huebner, E. A. (1991). *The home care and documentation guide: An orientation and resource manual for home health practitioners.* Gaithersburg, MD: Aspen.

Joint Commission on Accreditation of Healthcare Organizations (JCAHO). (1988a). *Home care standards for accreditation.* Chicago: Author.

Joint Commission on Accreditation of Healthcare Organizations (JCAHO). (1988b). *Monitoring and evaluation of the quality and appropriateness of care: A home care example.* Chicago: Author.

Kadushin, A. (1985). *Supervision in social work* (2nd ed.). New York: Columbia University Press.

Kane, N. M. (1989). The home care crisis of the nineties. *The Gerontologist, 29,* 24-31.

Kane, R. A. (1985). Assessing the elderly client. In A. Monk (Ed.), *Handbook of gerontological services* (pp. 43-69). New York: Van Nostrand Reinhold.

Kane, R. A. (1987). Comprehensive assessment. In G. L. Maddox (Ed.),*The encyclopedia of aging* (pp. 137-139). New York: Springer.

Kane, R. A., & Kane, R. L. (1981). *Assessing the elderly: A practical guide to measurement.* Lexington, MA: Lexington Books.

Kaye, L. W. (1982). Home care services for older people: An organizational analysis of provider experience. Final Report to the U.S. Department of Health and Human Services. OHDS-90-AT-0044/01.

Kaye, L. W. (1985a). Homecare. In A. Monk (Ed.), *Handbook of gerontological services* (pp. 408-432). New York: Van Nostrand Reinhold.

Kaye, L. W. (1985b). Home care for the aged: A fragile partnership. *Social Work, 30*(4), 312-317.

Kaye, L. W. (1986, June 9). Putting community services in perspective. Keynote address at the Professional Training Institute on "An Action Plan for Diversification" sponsored by the American Association of Homes and Services for the Aging, Chicago, IL.

Kaye, L. W. (1988, November 6). The evolution of private geriatric care management: Guidelines for responsible practice. Paper presented at the 4th annual conference of the National Association of Private Geriatric Care Managers, Philadelphia, PA.

Kaye, L. W. (1991). The future of community-based services for the old-old: Technological and ethical challenges. *Home Health Care Services Quarterly, 12*(1), 57-67.

Kaye, L. W., & Applegate, J. S. (1990). *Male caregivers to the elderly: Recognizing and aiding unrecognized family support.* Lexington, MA: Lexington Books.

Kaye, L. W., & Reisman, S. I. (1991a). *A comparative analysis of marketing strategies in health and human services for the elderly: Provider and consumer perspectives.* Bryn Mawr, PA: Bryn Mawr Graduate School of Social Work & Social Research.

Kaye, L. W., & Reisman, S. I. (1991b). Life prolongation technologies in home care for the frail elderly: Issues for training, policy, and research. *Journal of Gerontological Social Work, 16,* 79-91.

Kinderknecht, C. H. (1986, spring). In-home social work with abused or neglected elderly: An experiential guide to assessment and treatment. *Journal of Gerontological Social Work, 9*(3), 29-42.

Kirschner, C., & Rosengarten, L. (1982, November). The skilled social work role in home care. *Social Work,* 527-530.

Knight, B. (1986). *Psychotherapy with older adults.* Newbury Park, CA: Sage.

Kotler, P. (1980). *Marketing management: Analysis, planning and control.* Englewood Cliffs, NJ: Prentice-Hall.

Kranz, D. (1989). Demystifying home care quality assurance: A staff member's guide. *Journal of Home Health Care Practice, 3,* 1-9.

LaBarge, E. (1981). Counseling patients with senile dementia of the Alzheimer type and their families. *The Personnel and Guidance Journal,* 139-143.

Lawton, M. P. (1978). Institutions and alternatives for older people. *Health and Social Work, 3*(2), 108-134.

Lawton, M. P., Ward, M., & Yaffe, S. (1982). A research and service oriented multilevel assessment instrument. *Journal of Gerontology, 37*(1), 91-99.

Lee, J. T., & Stein, M. A. (1980). Eliminating duplication in home health care for the elderly: The Guale project. *Health and Social Work, 5*, 29-36.

Mace, N. L., & Rabins, P. V. (1981). *The 36-hour day.* Baltimore: Johns Hopkins University Press.

Macklin, R., & Callahan, D. (1990). Some examples to consider. In C. Zuckerman, N. N. Dubler, & B. Collopy (Eds.), *Home health care options: A guide for older persons and concerned families* (pp. 217-252). New York: Plenum.

MacStravic, R. (1977). *Marketing health care.* Rockville, MD: Aspen.

Martin, D. C., Morycz, R. K., McDowell, J., Snustad, D., & Karpf, M. (1985). Community-based geriatric assessment. *Journal of the American Geriatrics Society, 33*(9), 602-606.

McCann, A. R. (Ed.), (1987). *The annual clinical software guide for the human services: 1987.* New York: Brookdale Institute on Aging and Adult Human Development, Columbia University.

Meany-Handy, J. (1986). Marketing in home health care. In S. Stuart-Siddall (Ed.), *Home health care nursing: Administrative and clinical perspectives* (pp. 135-144). Rockville, MD: Aspen.

Monk, A. (1981). Social work with the aged: Principles of practice. *Social Work, 26*(1), 61-68.

Moore, F. M. (1988). *Homemaker-home health aide services: Policies and practices.* Owings Mills, MD: National Health Publishing.

Moore, F. M., & Layzer, E. (1983). Supporting the homemaker-home health aide as a valuable player on the home care team. *Pride Institute Journal of Long-Term Home Health Care, 2*, 19-23.

Moxley, D. P. (1989). *The practice of case management.* Newbury Park, CA: Sage.

Mundinger, M. O. (1983). *Home care controversy: Too little, too late, too costly.* Rockville, MD: Aspen.

Nassif, J. (1986a). *Homemaker-home health aide services for cancer patients and their families, a trainer's manual.* Washington, DC: National HomeCaring Council.

Nassif, J. (1986b). *Caring for cancer patients: A handbook for the homemaker-home health aide.* Washington, DC: National HomeCaring Council.

Nassif, J. (1986-1987, Winter). There's still no place like home: A primer on home health care. *Generations, XI*(2), 5-8.

Nassif, J. (1987). *Homemaker-home health aide services in support of high-tech patients and their families, a trainer's manual.* Washington, DC: National HomeCaring Council.

National Health Publishing. (1985). *Home health & hospice manual: Regulations and guidelines.* Owings Mill, MD: Rynd Communications.

National HomeCaring Council. (1982). *Supervision in home care.* New York: Author.

O'Brien, J. E., & Wagner, D. L. (1980). Help seeking by the frail elderly: problems in network analysis. *The Gerontologist, 20*(1), 78-83.

O'Malley, S. T. (1986). Reimbursement issues. In S. Stuart-Diddall (Ed.), *Home health care nursing: Administrative and clinical perspectives* (pp. 23-82) Rockville, MD: Aspen.

Parad, H. J. (Ed.). (1965). *Crisis intervention: Selected readings.* New York: Family Service Association of America.

Patton, M. Q. (1982). *Practical evaluation.* Beverly Hills, CA: Sage.

Pratt, C. C., Schmall, V. L., Wright, S., & Cleland, M. (1985). Burden and coping strategies of caregivers to Alzheimer's patients. *Family Relations, 34,* 27-33.

Randall, D. A. (1989). Legal liability in the home care setting: New technology and new risks. *Journal of Home Health Care Practice, 1* 27-35.

Rapoport, L. (1970). The state of crisis: Some theoretical considerations. In H. J. Parad (Ed.), *Crisis intervention: Selected readings.* New York: Family Service Association of America.

Reamer, F. G. (1987). Ethics committees in social work. *Social Work, 32,* 188-192.

Rossi, P. H., & Freeman, H. E. (1985). *Evaluation: A systematic approach.* Beverly Hills, CA: Sage.

Ryan, S. J., & Wassenberg, C. (1980). A hospital-based home care program. *Nursing Clinics of North America, 15*(2), 323-338.

Schmidt, G. L., & Keys, B. (1985). Group psychotherapy with family caregivers of demented. *The Gerontologist, 25,* 347-350.

Sherman, E. (1985). Casework services. In A. Monk (Ed.), *Handbook of gerontological services* (pp. 142-168). New York: Van Nostrand Reinhold.

Silverstone, B. (1981). Long-term care. *Health and Social Work, 6* (4), 28-34.

Silverstone, B., & Burack-Weiss, A. (1983a). The social work function in nursing homes and home care. In G. S. Getzel & M. J. Mellor (Eds.), *Gerontological social work practice in long-term care* (pp. 7-33). New York: Haworth.

Silverstone, B., & Burack-Weiss, A. (1983b). *Social work practice with the frail elderly and their families: The auxiliary function model.* Springfield, IL: Charles C Thomas.

Smith, M. J. (1990). *Program evaluation in the human services.* New York: Springer.

Spiegel, A. D. (1983). *Home healthcare.* Owings Mills, MD: National Health Publishing.

Spiegel, A. D., & Domanowski, G. (1983). Beginnings of home health care: A brief history. *PRIDE Institute Journal of Long Term Home Health Care, 2*(3), 28-33.

Steinberg, R. (1985). Access assistance and case management. In A. Monk (Ed.), *Handbook of gerontological services* (pp. 109-141). New York: Van Nostrand Reinhold.

Stuart-Siddall, S. (Ed.). (1986). *Home health care nursing: Administrative and clinical perspectives.* Rockville, MD: Aspen.

Tobin, S. S., & Toseland, R. (1985). Models of service for the elderly. In A. Monk (Ed.), *Handbook of gerontological services* (pp. 549-567). New York: Van Nostrand Reinhold.

Tonti, M. (1983). Working with the family. In B. Silverstone & A. Burke-Weiss (Eds.), *Social work practice with the frail elderly and their families: The auxiliary function model* (pp. 248-268). Springfield, IL: Charles C Thomas.

Tonti, M., & Silverstone, B. (1985). Services to families of the elderly. In A. Monk (Ed.), *Handbook of gerontological services* (pp. 211-239). New York: Van Nostrand Reinhold.

Trager, B. (1980, Spring). Home health care and national health policy. *Home Health Care Services Quarterly, 1*(2), 1-103.

Wasow, M. (1986). Support groups for family caregivers of patients with Alzheimer's disease. *Social Work, 37,* 93-97.

Weinstein, M. J., & Zlotnick, C. (1986). Project termination: Reintegration of demonstration clients into existing service systems. In A. O. Pelham & W. F. Clark (Eds.), *Managing home care for the elderly: Lessons from community-based agencies* (pp. 141-158). New York: Springer.

Wilson, S. J. (1980). *Recording: Guidelines for social workers.* New York: Free Press.

York, R. O. (1982). *Human service planning: Concepts, tools, & methods.* Chapel Hill, NC: The University of North Carolina Press.

Zarit, S. H., Reever, K. E., & Bach-Peterson, J. (1980). Relatives of the impaired elderly: Correlates of feelings of burden. *The Gerontologist, 20*(6), 646-655.

Author Index

Subject Index

About the Author

Lenard W. Kaye is Professor and Associate Dean at Bryn Mawr College Graduate School of Social Work & Social Research. He received his bachelor's degree at the State University of New York at Binghamton, his master's degree at New York University School of Social Work, and his doctorate at the Columbia University School of Social Work. He is the coauthor of *Resolving Grievances in the Nursing Home: A Study of the Ombudsman Program* and *Men as Caregivers to the Elderly: Understanding and Aiding Unrecognized Family Support* and the coeditor of *Congregate Housing for the Elderly: Theoretical, Policy, and Programmatic Perspectives.* He has published more than 60 book chapters and journal articles on issues in elder caregiving, long-term care advocacy, adult day care, home health care, retirement life-styles, and social work curriculum development.

Dr. Kaye sits on the editorial boards of the *Journal of Gerontological Social Work* and *Research on Social Work Practice*. He is a board member of numerous community organizations, the Past President of the New York State Society on Aging and of Understanding Aging, Inc., and a Fellow of the Gerontological Society of America. He has conducted recent research in the area of older adult, part-time subsidized employment and is currently completing a book on marketing techniques in health and social services for the aged. His current research is in the areas of self-help support groups for older women and the ethical and legal aspects of high technology home care.